Specker

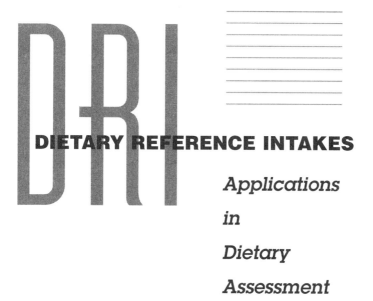

DIETARY REFERENCE INTAKES

Applications

in

Dietary

Assessment

A Report of the
Subcommittee on Interpretation and
Uses of Dietary Reference Intakes and
the Standing Committee on the Scientific Evaluation of
Dietary Reference Intakes

Food and Nutrition Board

INSTITUTE OF MEDICINE

D0778372

NATIONAL ACADEMY PRESS
Washington, D.C.

NATIONAL ACADEMY PRESS • 2101 Constitution Avenue, N.W. • Washington, DC 20418

NOTICE: The project that is the subject of this report was approved by the Governing Board of the National Research Council, whose members are drawn from the councils of the National Academy of Sciences, the National Academy of Engineering, and the Institute of Medicine. The members of the committee responsible for the report were chosen for their special competences and with regard for appropriate balance.

Support for this project was provided by Health Canada; U.S. Department of Health and Human Services Office of Disease Prevention and Health Promotion, Contract No. 282-96-0033; the Dietary Reference Intakes Private Foundation Fund, including the Dannon Institute and the International Life Sciences Institute; and the Dietary Reference Intakes Corporate Donors' Fund. Contributors to the Fund to date include Daiichi Fine Chemicals, Inc.; Kemin Foods, L.C.; M&M/Mars; Mead Johnson Nutritionals; Nabisco Foods Group; Natural Source Vitamin E Association; Roche Vitamins Inc.; U.S. Borax; and Weider Nutritional Group. The opinions or conclusions expressed herein are those of the committee and do not necessarily reflect those of the funders.

Library of Congress Cataloging-in-Publication Data

Dietary reference intakes. Applications in dietary assessment : a report of the Subcommittees on Interpretation and Uses of Dietary Reference Intakes and Upper Reference Levels of Nutrients, and the Standing Committee on the Scientific Evaluation of Dietary Reference Intakes, Food and Nutrition Board, Institute of Medicine.
    p. ; cm.
Includes bibliographical references and index.
ISBN 0-309-07311-1 (hardcover) — ISBN 0-309-07183-6 (pbk.)
  1. Nutrition. 2. Reference values (Medicine) 3. Nutrition—Evaluation. I. Title: Applications in dietary assessment. II. Institute of Medicine (U.S.). Subcommittee on Interpretation and Uses of Dietary Reference Intakes. III. Institute of Medicine (U.S.). Subcommittee on Upper Reference Levels of Nutrients. IV. Institute of Medicine (U.S.). Standing Committee on the Scientific Evaluation of Dietary Reference Intakes.
  [DNLM: 1. Nutrition Assessment. 2. Dietetics. 3. Nutrition Policy. 4. Nutritional Requirements. QU 146 D5656 2001]
QP141 .D525 2001
613.2—dc21

00-069187

This report is available for sale from the National Academy Press, 2101 Constitution Avenue, N.W., Box 285, Washington, DC 20055; call (800) 624-6242 or (202) 334-3313 (in the Washington metropolitan area), or visit the NAP's on-line bookstore at **http://www.nap.edu**.

For more information about the Institute of Medicine or the Food and Nutrition Board, visit the IOM home page at **http://www.iom.edu.**

"Knowing is not enough; we must apply.
Willing is not enough; we must do."
—Goethe

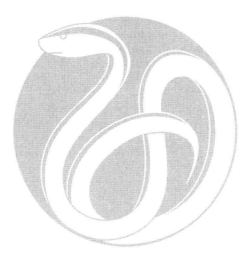

INSTITUTE OF MEDICINE

Shaping the Future for Health

THE NATIONAL ACADEMIES

National Academy of Sciences
National Academy of Engineering
Institute of Medicine
National Research Council

The **National Academy of Sciences** is a private, nonprofit, self-perpetuating society of distinguished scholars engaged in scientific and engineering research, dedicated to the furtherance of science and technology and to their use for the general welfare. Upon the authority of the charter granted to it by the Congress in 1863, the Academy has a mandate that requires it to advise the federal government on scientific and technical matters. Dr. Bruce M. Alberts is president of the National Academy of Sciences.

The **National Academy of Engineering** was established in 1964, under the charter of the National Academy of Sciences, as a parallel organization of outstanding engineers. It is autonomous in its administration and in the selection of its members, sharing with the National Academy of Sciences the responsibility for advising the federal government. The National Academy of Engineering also sponsors engineering programs aimed at meeting national needs, encourages education and research, and recognizes the superior achievements of engineers. Dr. William A. Wulf is president of the National Academy of Engineering.

The **Institute of Medicine** was established in 1970 by the National Academy of Sciences to secure the services of eminent members of appropriate professions in the examination of policy matters pertaining to the health of the public. The Institute acts under the responsibility given to the National Academy of Sciences by its congressional charter to be an adviser to the federal government and, upon its own initiative, to identify issues of medical care, research, and education. Dr. Kenneth I. Shine is president of the Institute of Medicine.

The **National Research Council** was organized by the National Academy of Sciences in 1916 to associate the broad community of science and technology with the Academy's purposes of furthering knowledge and advising the federal government. Functioning in accordance with general policies determined by the Academy, the Council has become the principal operating agency of both the National Academy of Sciences and the National Academy of Engineering in providing services to the government, the public, and the scientific and engineering communities. The Council is administered jointly by both Academies and the Institute of Medicine. Dr. Bruce M. Alberts and Dr. William A. Wulf are chairman and vice chairman, respectively, of the National Research Council.

SUBCOMMITTEE ON INTERPRETATION AND USES OF DIETARY REFERENCE INTAKES

SUZANNE P. MURPHY *(Chair)*, Cancer Research Center of Hawaii, University of Hawaii, Honolulu

LENORE ARAB, Department of Epidemiology, University of North Carolina School of Public Health, Chapel Hill

SUSAN I. BARR, Faculty of Agricultural Sciences, University of British Columbia, Vancouver

SUSAN T. BORRA, International Food Information Council, Washington, D.C.

ALICIA L. CARRIQUIRY, Department of Statistics, Iowa State University, Ames

BARBARA L. DEVANEY, Mathematica Policy Research, Princeton, New Jersey

JOHANNA T. DWYER, Frances Stern Nutrition Center, New England Medical Center and Tufts University, Boston, Massachusetts

JEAN-PIERRE HABICHT, Division of Nutritional Sciences, Cornell University, Ithaca, New York

JANET C. KING,* USDA Western Human Nutrition Research Center, University of California, Davis

HARRIET V. KUHNLEIN, Centre for Indigenous Peoples' Nutrition and Environment, McGill University, Ste. Anne de Bellevue, Quebec

Consultant

GEORGE BEATON, GHB Consulting, Willowdale, Ontario

Staff

Mary Poos, Study Director
Alice L. Vorosmarti, Research Associate
Michele Ramsey, Senior Project Assistant
Karah Nazor, Project Assistant

*Term of Service
February 17, 1998, to June 30, 1999

v

SUBCOMMITTEE ON UPPER REFERENCE LEVELS OF NUTRIENTS

Preface

This report is one of a series that relates to the development of Dietary Reference Intakes. This report focuses on applications of Dietary Reference Intakes (DRIs) in dietary assessment from the Subcommittee on Interpretation and Uses of Dietary Reference Intakes (Uses Subcommittee) of the Standing Committee on the Scientific Evaluation of Dietary Reference Intakes (DRI Committee). A forthcoming report from this Subcommittee will address applications of DRIs in dietary planning.

The Food and Nutrition Board anticipated that considerable guidance would be needed to assist American and Canadian health professionals in the transition from using the former Recommended Dietary Allowances (RDAs) for the United States and Recommended Nutrient Intakes (RNIs) for Canada to using the new DRIs, and thus charged the DRI Committee and the Uses Subcommittee to develop advice on the appropriate uses of these new references.

In the past, RDAs and RNIs were the primary values that were available to health professionals for planning and assessing the diets of individuals and groups. However, the former RDAs and RNIs were not ideally suited for many of these applications. The new DRIs represent a more complete set of values that were developed anticipating diverse uses for planning and/or assessment and thus allow more robust approaches. To assist health professionals in their use of the new DRIs, the Uses Subcommittee divided its work into two parts: the current report examines the appropriate use of each of the available DRI values in *assessing* nutrient intakes of groups and of individuals and a second report will present information on the appropriate use of specific DRI values in the *planning* of diets for groups and for individuals. Each report will present the statistical underpinnings for the various uses of the DRI values, present sample applications, and provide guidelines to help professionals determine when specific uses are inappropriate.

A probability approach to assessing prevalence of nutrient inadequacy in groups was developed and presented—with extensive statistical validation and identification of sources of error—in the National Research Council Report, *Nutrient Adequacy* (NRC, 1986). The availability of Estimated Average Requirements (EARs), one of the categories of DRIs, makes the use of the probability approach possible. A modified approach, using the Estimated Average Requirement (EAR) as a cutpoint for assessing the prevalence of nutrient inadequacy in groups, is presented in this report. The cut-point method, however, is not a new independent approach; it is a modification of the probability approach. The statistical validation of the EAR cut-point method to assess prevalence of inadequacy in groups is presented in this report.

When the initial plan to revise the former RDAs was published (IOM, 1994), the Food and Nutrition Board envisioned the simultaneous establishment of the DRI Committee and two standing subcommittees, the Subcommittee on Upper Reference Intake Levels of Nutrients and the Uses Subcommittee. However, circumstances precluded the early convening of the Uses Subcommittee. It was not established until early 1998, after the release of the first two nutrient reports (IOM, 1997, 1998b).

The Uses Subcommittee, with expertise in nutrition, dietetics, statistics, nutritional epidemiology, public health, economics, and consumer perspectives, was charged to review the scientific literature regarding the uses of dietary reference standards and their applications, and to provide guidance for (1) the appropriate application of DRIs for specific purposes and identification of inappropriate applications, (2) appropriate assumptions regarding intake and requirement distributions, (3) adjustments needed to minimize potential errors in dietary intake data, and (4) appropriate use of DRI values of specific nutrients. Starting with the report of the Panel on Dietary Antioxidants and Related Compounds, this specific guidance will be found in the nutrient reports.

This report reflects the work of the Food and Nutrition Board's DRI Committee, the Uses Subcommittee, and the Subcommittee on Upper Reference Levels of Nutrients. The support of the government of Canada and Canadian scientists in establishing the Uses Subcommittee represents a pioneering first step in the standardization of nutrient reference intakes in North America. A brief description of the overall DRI project is given in Appendix A.

This report has been reviewed by individuals chosen for their diverse perspectives and technical expertise, in accordance with procedures approved by the National Research Council's Report Review Committee. The purpose of this independent review was to provide candid and critical comments to assist the authors and the Institute of Medicine in making the published report as sound as possible and to ensure that the report meets institutional standards for objectivity, evidence, and responsiveness to the study charge. The contents of the review comments and draft manuscript remain confidential to protect the integrity of the deliberative process.

We wish to thank the following individuals for their participation in the review of this report: Cynthia M. Beall, Ph.D., Case Western Reserve University; William H. Danforth, M.D., Washington University; Mary J. Kretsch, Ph.D., RD, U.S. Department of Agriculture; George P. McCabe, Ph.D., Purdue University; Grace L. Ostenso, Ph.D., Washington, D.C.; Eric B. Rimm, Sc.D., Harvard School of Public Health; Christopher P. Sempos. Ph.D., State University of New York; Helen Smiciklas-Wright, Ph.D., RD, Pennsylvania State University; Paul D. Stolley, M.D., MPH, University of Maryland at Baltimore; and Valerie Tarasuk, Ph.D., University of Toronto.

Although the individuals listed above provided many constructive comments and suggestions, responsibility for the final content of this report rests solely with the authoring committee and the Institute of Medicine.

The DRI Committee wishes to acknowledge, in particular, the commitment and dedication shown by Suzanne P. Murphy, chair of the Uses Subcommittee. Dr. Murphy's expertise and direction were key to the resolution of controversial issues and to the presentation of technically complex information and its statistical basis in a clear and readily understandable manner. Sincere thanks are also extended to George H. Beaton for his willingness to participate as a technical consultant to the Uses Subcommittee. His provocative comments and assistance provided an important impetus to move the conceptual framework, while still in development and far from complete, forward. Not all issues have been resolved, but the foundation has been initiated. We also extend special thanks to the staff of the Food and Nutrition Board and especially to Mary Poos, study director for the Uses Subcommittee, for her many contributions to the synthesis of the report. We recognize the significant efforts of the Subcommittee and the Food and Nutrition Board staff that were required to achieve the completion of this report. It is, of course,

the Food and Nutrition Board staff who get much of the work completed, so on behalf of the DRI Committee and the Board, we wish
to thank Allison Yates, Director of the Food and Nutrition Board
and study director for the DRI activity, for her continued oversight,
and also recognize, with appreciation, the contributions of Michele
Ramsey, Alice Vorosmarti, Karah Nazor, Sandra Schlicker, and Gail
Spears. We wish also to thank Carol Suitor for scientific and organi-
zational review, Judith Dickson for editing the manuscript, and Mike
Edington and Claudia Carl for assistance with its publication.

Vernon Young
Chair, Standing Committee on the Scientific
Evaluation of Dietary Reference Intakes

Cutberto Garza
Chair, Food and Nutrition Board

Contents

Summary

This report is one of a series designed to provide guidance on the interpretation and uses of Dietary Reference Intakes (DRIs). The term *Dietary Reference Intakes* is relatively new to the field of nutrition and refers to a set of four nutrient-based reference values that can be used for assessing and planning diets and for many other purposes. Specifically, this report provides guidance to nutrition and health professionals for applications of the DRIs in dietary *assessment* of individuals and groups. It also demonstrates that these uses of the DRIs are based on what is reasonable from a statistical as well as nutritional point of view. The report encourages nutritional evaluation from a quantitative perspective and in this regard follows the 1986 National Research Council report on nutrient adequacy by providing the theoretical underpinnings of the various methods discussed. The report emphasizes that dietary assessment of either groups or individuals must be based on an estimate of usual (long-term) intake. In a departure from many of the more traditional analyses, the use of standard deviations to estimate uncertainty is emphasized. It is hoped that this use of standard deviations of estimates of usual intake, nutrient inadequacy, nutrient requirements, or any other parameter of interest will become the norm in nutritional analyses.

Throughout this report the Subcommittee on Interpretation and Uses of Dietary Reference Intakes distinguishes between methods of evaluating the nutrient intakes of individuals (Chapter 3), and methods for evaluating the intakes of groups (Chapters 4–7), as these are two very different applications. A subsequent report will

1

address appropriate uses of the DRIs for *planning* diets of groups and individuals.

THE CONCEPT OF DIETARY REFERENCE STANDARDS

In 1941, the Food and Nutrition Board first proposed the Recommended Dietary Allowance (RDA) for the U.S. population "to serve as a goal for good nutrition and as a 'yardstick' by which to measure progress toward that goal..." (NRC, 1941, p. 1). Even today, the many specific uses and applications of dietary reference standards fall into the two general categories defined implicitly in 1941: diet assessment and planning. Diet assessment applications involve determining the probable adequacy or inadequacy of observed intakes (a yardstick by which to measure progress). Diet planning applications involve using dietary reference standards to develop recommendations for what food intakes should be (as a goal for good nutrition). Obviously, these two general applications are interrelated.

The first dietary standards in Canada were issued by the Canadian Council on Nutrition in 1938. At the time it was stated that the standards were to be used as the basis for evaluating observed diets. In 1942, rather than revise the 1938 standards, the Canadian Council on Nutrition recommended that the 1941 RDAs be applied in Canada. However, by 1945 differences in the approach of the Canadian Daily Recommended Nutrient Intakes (DRNIs) and U.S. standards had become evident. The differences were conceptual and related to the application of the standards to individuals versus application to groups.

The most recent versions of the Canadian (now shortened to Recommended Nutrient Intakes [RNIs]) (Health and Welfare Canada, 1990) and U.S. (NRC, 1989) standards did not differ in the described derivations of the recommended intakes but some differences remained in how intended uses were described.

WHAT ARE DIETARY REFERENCE INTAKES?

The new Dietary Reference Intakes (DRIs) differ from the former Recommended Dietary Allowances (RDAs) and Recommended Nutrient Intakes (RNIs) conceptually. These differences are that: (1) where specific data on safety and efficacy exist, reduction in the risk of chronic degenerative disease is included in the formulation of the recommendation rather than just the absence of signs of deficiency; (2) upper levels of intake are established where data exist regarding risk of adverse health effects; and (3) components of food that may not meet the traditional concept of a nutrient but are of possible benefit to health will be reviewed, and if sufficient data exist, reference intakes will be established.

Where adequate information is available, each nutrient has a set of DRIs. A nutrient has either an Estimated Average Requirement (EAR) and an RDA, or an Adequate Intake (AI). When an EAR for the nutrient cannot be determined (and therefore, neither can the RDA), then an AI is set for the nutrient. In addition, many nutrients have a Tolerable Upper Intake Level (UL). A brief definition of each of the DRIs is presented in Box S-1.

Like the former RDAs and RNIs, each DRI refers to the average daily nutrient intake of apparently healthy individuals over time. The amount of intake may vary substantially from day to day without ill effect in most cases.

The chosen criterion of nutritional adequacy or adverse effect on which the DRI is based is different for each nutrient and is identified in the DRI nutrient reports. In some cases the criterion for a nutrient may differ for individuals at different life stages. In developing recommendations, emphasis is placed on the reasons underlying the particular criterion of adequacy used to establish the requirement for each nutrient. This requirement is typically presented as a single number for various life stage and gender groups rather than as multiple endpoints even if the criterion of adequacy for the end-

---

Box S-1 Dietary Reference Intakes

Estimated Average Requirement (EAR): the average daily nutrient intake level estimated to meet the requirement of half the healthy individuals in a particular life stage and gender group.

Recommended Dietary Allowance (RDA): the average daily nutrient intake level sufficient to meet the nutrient requirement of nearly all (97 to 98 percent) healthy individuals in a particular life stage and gender group.

Adequate Intake (AI): a recommended average daily nutrient intake level based on observed or experimentally determined approximations or estimates of nutrient intake by a group (or groups) of apparently healthy people that are assumed to be adequate—used when an RDA cannot be determined.

Tolerable Upper Intake Level (UL): the highest average daily nutrient intake level likely to pose no risk of adverse health effects to almost all individuals in the general population. As intake increases above the UL, the potential risk of adverse effects increases.

point differs. A more detailed discussion of the origin and framework of the DRIs is presented in Appendix A. Recommended intakes for the nutrients examined to date are presented at the end of this book.

The introduction of multiple dietary reference intakes—the EAR, RDA, AI, and UL—requires that applications for each be carefully developed and clearly explained. Box S-2 provides a brief introduction to appropriate uses of the DRIs for assessment, but it lacks the detail needed for their application (see Chapters 3–7).

Various professionals applying the former RDAs and RNIs—nutrition researchers, policy makers, nutrition educators, epidemiologists, and many others—may need guidance in using and interpreting

---

Box S-2 Uses of DRIs for Assessing Intakes of Individuals and Groups

For an Individual

EAR: use to examine the probability that usual intake is inadequate.

RDA: usual intake at or above this level has a low probability of inadequacy.

AI: usual intake at or above this level has a low probability of inadequacy.

UL: usual intake above this level may place an individual at risk of adverse effects from excessive nutrient intake.

For a Group

EAR: use to estimate the prevalence of inadequate intakes within a group.

RDA: do not use to assess intakes of groups.

AI: mean usual intake at or above this level implies a low prevalence of inadequate intakes.[a]

UL: use to estimate the percentage of the population at potential risk of adverse effects from excessive nutrient intake.

EAR = Estimated Average Requirement
RDA = Recommended Dietary Allowance
AI = Adequate Intake
UL = Tolerable Upper Intake Level

[a]When the AI for a nutrient is not based on mean intakes of healthy populations, this assessment is made with less confidence.

the new DRI values. This report is aimed at meeting this need as well as providing the theoretical background and statistical justification for application of the DRIs in the area of dietary assessment.

USING DRIs TO ASSESS NUTRIENT INTAKES OF INDIVIDUALS

It can be appropriate to compare intakes of individuals with specific Dietary Reference Intakes (DRIs), even though dietary intake data alone cannot be used to ascertain an individual's nutritional status. Dietary assessment is one component of a nutritional status assessment, provided that accurate dietary intake data are collected, the correct DRI is selected for the assessment, and the results are interpreted appropriately. Ideally, intake data are combined with clinical, biochemical, and anthropometric information to provide a valid assessment of an individual's nutritional status.

Using the EAR to Assess Individuals

Assessing individual diets for apparent nutrient adequacy addresses the following question, Given an individual's observed intakes on a small number of days, is that individual's usual nutrient intake adequate or not? Comparing an individual's intake to his or her requirement for a nutrient is difficult because: (1) a given individual's actual *requirement* is not known; and (2) it is seldom possible to measure an individual's long-term *usual intake* of the nutrient due to day-to-day variation in intake and intake measurement errors. Theoretically, the probability of inadequacy can be calculated for an individual's usual nutrient intake using the EAR and standard deviation of requirement. However, since an individual's usual intake is almost never known, a statistical approach is suggested in Chapter 3 and Appendix B that allows an evaluation of *observed intake* and an estimation of the confidence one has that usual intake is above (or below) an individual's requirement, based on the observed intake. This approach is based on the following assumptions:

- The Estimated Average Requirement (EAR) is the best estimate of an individual's requirement.
- There is person-to-person variation in the requirement. The standard deviation of the requirement is an indicator of how much the individual's requirement for a nutrient can deviate from the median requirement (EAR) in the population.
- Mean observed intake of an individual is the best estimate of an

individual's usual intake.

• There is day-to-day variation in intake for an individual. The within-person standard deviation of intakes is an indicator of how much observed intake may deviate from usual intake.

Inferences about the adequacy of an individual's diet can be made by looking at the difference between observed intake and the median requirement. If this difference is large and positive, that is, if observed intake is much greater than the median requirement, then it is likely that an individual's intake is adequate. Conversely, if the difference is large and negative, that is, observed intake is much less than the median requirement, then it is likely that an individual's intake is not adequate. In between there is considerable uncertainty about the adequacy of the individual's intake.

For practical purposes, many users of the DRIs may find it useful to consider that observed intakes below the EAR very likely need to be improved (because the probability of adequacy is 50 percent or less), and those between the EAR and the Recommended Dietary Allowance (RDA) probably need to be improved (because the probability of adequacy is less than 97 to 98 percent). Only if intakes have been observed for a large number of days and are at or above the RDA, or observed intakes for fewer days are well above the RDA, should one have a high level of confidence that the intake is adequate. It is hoped that computer software will be developed that will determine these probabilities (as described in Appendix B), thus offering more objective alternatives when individual intakes are evaluated.

Using the AI to Assess Individuals

Some nutrients have an Adequate Intake (AI) because the evidence was not sufficient to establish an EAR and thus an RDA for the nutrient in question. The approach described above for the EAR cannot be used for nutrients that have an AI. However, a statistically based hypothesis testing procedure for comparing observed intake to the AI may be used. This is a simple z-test, which is constructed using the standard deviation of daily intake of the nutrient.

What conclusions can be drawn about the adequacy of individual intakes for nutrients with AIs? First, if an individual's usual intake equals or exceeds the AI, it can be concluded that the diet is almost certainly adequate. If, however, their intake falls below the AI, no quantitative (or qualitative) estimate can be made of the probability of nutrient inadequacy. Professional judgment, based on additional types of information about the individual, should be exercised when interpreting intakes below the AI.

Using the UL to Assess Individuals

Assessing individual diets for risk of adverse effects from excessive intake addresses the question, Given an individual's observed intake on a small number of days, is that individual's usual nutrient intake so high that it poses a risk of adverse health effects? The answer is obtained by comparing usual intake to the Tolerable Upper Intake Level (UL). A hypothesis test similar to the one proposed above for the AI can be used to decide whether usual intake is below the UL. For some nutrients, the intake to be considered is from supplements, fortificants, and medications only, while for other nutrients one may need to consider intake from food as well.

The UL is set at the highest level that is likely to pose no risk of adverse health effects for almost all individuals in the general population, including sensitive individuals; but it is not possible to know who is most sensitive. If usual intake exceeds the UL, it may pose a risk for some healthy individuals. The consequences of nutrient excess are much more severe for some nutrients than for others, and for some nutrients the consequences may be irreversible.

The Bottom Line: Assessing Individual Diets

In all cases the individual's true requirement and usual intake can only be approximated. Thus, assessment of dietary adequacy for an individual is imprecise and must be interpreted cautiously in combination with other types of information about the individual.

USING DRIs TO ASSESS NUTRIENT INTAKES OF GROUPS

What proportion of the group has a usual intake of a nutrient that is less than their requirement for the same nutrient? This is one of the most basic questions that can be asked about nutritional needs of a group, and is critically important from a public health perspective. Clearly, the implications are different if 30 versus 3 percent of individuals are estimated to be inadequate. Another basic question is, What proportion of the group has a usual intake of a nutrient so high that it places them at risk of adverse health effects?

The assessment of intake of groups requires obtaining accurate data on intake, selecting the appropriate Dietary Reference Intakes (DRIs), adjusting intake distributions for within-person variability and survey-related effects, and interpreting the results appropriately. Assessment of groups for the adequacy of intake also involves choosing between two methods: (1) the probability approach or (2) the Estimated Average Requirement (EAR) cut-point method. Both are presented in detail in Chapter 4.

Individuals in a group vary both in the amounts of a nutrient they consume and in their requirements for the nutrient. If information were available on both the usual intakes and the requirements of all individuals in a group, determining the proportion of the group with intakes less than their requirements would be straightforward. One would simply observe how many individuals had inadequate intakes. Unfortunately, collecting such data is impractical. Therefore, rather than actually observing prevalence of inadequate intakes in the group, it can only be approximated by using other methods.

Using the EAR to Assess Groups

Regardless of the method chosen to actually estimate the prevalence of inadequacy, the EAR is the appropriate DRI to use when assessing the adequacy of group intakes. To demonstrate the pivotal importance of the EAR in assessing groups, the probability approach and the EAR cut-point method are described briefly below.

The Probability Approach

The probability approach is a statistical method that combines the distributions of requirements and intakes in the group to produce an estimate of the expected proportion of individuals at risk for inadequacy (NRC, 1986). For this method to perform well, little or no correlation should exist between intakes and requirements in the group. The concept is simple: at very low intakes the risk of inadequacy is high, whereas at very high intakes the risk of inadequacy is negligible. In fact, with information about the distribution of requirements in the group (median, variance, and shape), a value for risk of inadequacy can be attached to each intake level. Because there is a range of usual intakes in a group, the prevalence of inadequacy—the average group risk—is estimated as the weighted average of the risks at each possible intake level. Thus, the probability approach combines the two distributions: the requirement distribution which provides the risk of inadequacy at each intake level, and the usual intake distribution which provides the intake levels for the group and the frequency of each.

To compute the risk to attach to each intake level, one needs to know the EAR (the median) of the requirement distribution as well as its variance and its shape. Without an EAR, the probability approach cannot be used to estimate the prevalence of inadequacy.

The EAR Cut-Point Method

With some additional assumptions, a simpler version of the probability approach can be applied with essentially the same success. The EAR cut-point method can be used if no correlation exists between intakes and requirements (as in the probability approach above), if the distribution of requirements can be assumed to be symmetrical around the EAR, and if the variance of intakes is greater than the variance of requirements. Table S-1 indicates whether these conditions have been met for nutrients for which DRIs have been determined at the time of publication.

The EAR cut-point method is simpler because rather than estimating the risk of inadequacy for each individual's intake level, one simply counts how many individuals in the group of interest have usual intakes that are below the EAR. That proportion is the estimate of the proportion of individuals in the group with inadequate intakes. (For a theoretical justification of this simplified cut-point method, see Chapter 4 or Appendixes C and D.)

Adjusting Intake Distributions

Regardless of the method chosen to assess prevalence of inadequate nutrient intakes in a group of individuals, information is required about the distribution of usual intakes of the nutrient in the group. The distribution of those usual intakes in the group is referred to as the *usual intake distribution* or the *adjusted intake distribution*. Adjustments to the distribution of observed intakes are needed to partially remove the day-to-day variability in intakes (within-person variation). The resulting estimated usual intake distribution of a dietary component should then better reflect the individual-to-individual variation of intakes of that component within the group.

Usual intake distributions can be estimated by statistically adjusting the distribution of intake of each individual in the group. This general approach was proposed by NRC (1986) and was further developed by Nusser et al. (1996). To adjust intake distributions, it is necessary to have at least two independent days of dietary intake data for a representative subsample of individuals in the group (or at least three days when data are collected over consecutive days).

TABLE S-1 Summary of Dietary Reference Intakes (DRIs) for Nutrients and Assumptions Necessary to Apply the Estimated Average Requirement (EAR) Cut-Point Method for Assessing the Prevalence of Inadequacy for Groups

	Established DRIs[a]			
Nutrient	EAR	RDA	AI	UL
Magnesium	+	+		+
Phosphorus	+	+		+
Selenium	+	+		+
Thiamin	+	+		
Riboflavin	+	+		
Niacin	+	+		+
Vitamin B$_6$	+	+		+
Folate	+	+		+
Vitamin B$_{12}$	+	+		
Vitamin C	+	+		+
Vitamin E	+	+		+
Calcium			+	+
Fluoride			+	+
Biotin			+	
Choline			+	+
Vitamin D			+	+
Pantothenic Acid			+	

[a] RDA = Recommended Dietary Allowance; AI = Adequate Intake, cannot be used with the cut-point method; UL = Tolerable Upper Intake Level.

[b] Due to little information on the variance of requirements, published DRIs have assumed a coefficient of variation (CV) of 10 percent unless data for a specific nutrient demonstrate a greater variability. Variance of intake, as calculated from the 1994–1996

If intake distributions are not properly adjusted both for within-person variation and survey-related effects such as interview method and interview sequence, the prevalence of nutrient inadequacy will be incorrectly estimated no matter which of the methods discussed earlier is chosen. If only one day of intake data is available for each individual in the sample, it may still be possible to adjust the observed intake distribution by using an estimate of within-person variation in intakes estimated from other data sets.

Meets the Assumptions of the Cut-Point Method

Variance of Intake is Greater than Variance of Requirement[b]	Requirement Distributions Symmetrical[c]	Intake and Requirement Independent or Have Low Correlation	Coefficient of Variance of the Requirement Estimate[d] (%)
Yes	Assumed	Yes	10
Yes	Assumed	Yes	10
Yes	Assumed	Yes	10
Yes	Assumed	Yes	10
Yes	Assumed	Yes	10
Yes	Assumed	Yes	15
Yes	Assumed	Yes	10
Yes	Assumed	Yes	10
Yes	Assumed	Yes	10
Yes	Assumed	Yes	10
Yes	Assumed	Yes	10

Continuing Survey of Food Intake by Individuals, indicates that for all nutrients intake variance is well above the assumed requirement variance.
[c] Data to determine the shape of requirement distributions are lacking for most nutrients; therefore, symmetry is assumed unless there are adequate data indicating otherwise.
[d] The CV of the requirement estimate is needed for the probability approach.

Using the RDA Is Inappropriate for Assessing Groups

The Recommended Dietary Allowance (RDA), by definition, is an intake level that exceeds the requirements of 97 to 98 percent of all individuals when requirements in the group have a normal distribution. Thus, the RDA should not be used as a cut-point for assessing nutrient intakes of groups because a serious overestimation of the proportion of the group at risk of inadequacy would result.

Using the Mean Intake Is Inappropriate for Assessing Groups

Mean or median intake seldom, if ever, can be used to assess nutrient adequacy of group diets. In the past, nutrient intake data have frequently been evaluated by comparing mean intakes with RDAs. In particular, studies that found mean intakes equal to or exceeding the RDA often concluded that group diets were adequate and conformed to recognized nutritional standards. However, this is inappropriate because the prevalence of inadequacy depends on the shape and variation of the usual intake distribution, not on mean intake. Indeed, for most nutrients, group mean intake must exceed the RDA for there to be an acceptably low prevalence of inadequate intakes. Moreover, the greater the variability in usual intake relative to the variability in requirement, the greater the mean usual intake must be relative to the RDA to ensure that only a small proportion of the group has inadequate intake. If group mean intake equals the RDA, there will be a substantial proportion of the group with usual intake less than requirement. Chapter 4 provides more detail on issues related to comparing mean intakes to the DRIs. Even stronger caution is needed when comparing group mean intakes with the EAR. If mean intake equals the EAR, it is likely that a very high proportion of the population will have inadequate usual intake. In fact, roughly half of the population is expected to have intakes less than their requirement (except for energy).

Using the AI to Assess Groups

When the AI represents the group mean intake of an apparently healthy group (or groups) of people, similar groups with mean intakes at or above the AI can be assumed to have a low prevalence of inadequate intakes for the defined criteria of nutritional status. For AIs that were either experimentally derived or developed from a combination of experimental and intake data, a similar assessment can be made, but with less confidence. Each AI is described in terms of its derivation and selected criterion of adequacy in the individual nutrient panel reports (IOM, 1997, 1998b, 2000). When mean intakes of groups are below the AI it is not possible to make any assumptions about the extent of intake inadequacy. It is not appropriate to try to estimate an EAR from an AI.

Using the UL to Assess Groups

The Tolerable Upper Intake Level (UL) is the appropriate DRI to use to assess the risk of adverse health effects from excessive nutrient intake. As intake increases above the UL, the potential for risk of adverse health effects increases.

Depending on the nutrient, the UL assessment requires accurate information on usual daily intake from all sources, or from supplements, fortificants, and medications only. Usual intake distributions will allow determination of the fraction of the population exceeding the UL. This fraction may be at risk of adverse health effects.

Difficulties arise in attempts to quantify the risk (likelihood) of adverse health effects in the general population from daily nutrient intakes exceeding the UL. The use of uncertainty factors to arrive at the UL reflects inaccuracies in reported nutrient intake data, uncertainties in the dose-response data on adverse health effects, extrapolation of data from animal experiments, severity of the adverse effect, and variation in individual susceptibility. As more accurate data from human studies become available, predicting the magnitude of the risk associated with intakes exceeding the UL may become possible. For now it is advisable to use the UL as a cutoff for safe intake.

Applications in Group Assessment

The evaluation of dietary survey data merits special attention. This includes three major components: describing the dietary survey data, estimating the prevalence of inadequate or excessive intake, and evaluating differences among subgroups in intake. These applications are discussed in Chapter 7 and summarized in Table S-2.

Bottom Line: Assessing Group Intakes

Dietary assessment at the group level typically involves comparing usual nutrient intakes with nutrient requirements to assess the prevalence of nutrient inadequacy. The preferred outcome measure used to assess the prevalence of inadequate nutrient intake is the percentage of a group with usual intake less than the EAR. For nutrients with an AI, the best that can be done is to look at mean and median intake relative to the AI. However, when mean intakes of groups are less than the AI, nothing can be inferred about the prevalence of inadequacy. To estimate the proportion of the population at risk of excessive intake, the outcome measure is the per-

TABLE S-2 Applications: Evaluating Dietary Survey Data

Measures	Nutrients
What are the characteristics of the distribution of usual nutrient intake?	
Mean usual nutrient intake Median usual nutrient intake Percentiles of usual nutrient intake distribution	All nutrients under consideration
What proportion of the population has inadequate usual nutrient intake?	

Percentage with usual intake less than
  the Estimated Average Requirement
  (EAR)
	Vitamins: thiamin, riboflavin, niacin,
	  B_6, folate, B_{12}, C, and E
	Elements: phosphorus, magnesium,
	  selenium

What proportion of the population is at potential risk of adverse effects?	

Percentage with usual intake greater
  than the Tolerable Upper Intake
  Level (UL)
	Vitamins: niacin, B_6, folate, choline,
	  C, D, and E
	Elements: calcium, phosphorus,
	  magnesium, fluoride, selenium

Are there differences in nutrient intakes and differences in nutrient adequacy for different subgroups of the population?	

Mean usual nutrient intake for
  subgroups
Median usual nutrient intake for
  subgroups
Percentiles of the usual nutrient
  intake distribution for subgroups
	All nutrients under consideration

Percentage with usual intake less
  than the EAR for subgroups
	Vitamins: thiamin, riboflavin, niacin,
	  B_6, folate, B_{12}, C, and E
	Elements: phosphorus, magnesium,
	  selenium

Percentage with usual intake
  greater than the UL for subgroups
	Vitamins: niacin, B_6, folate, choline,
	  C, D, and E
	Elements: calcium, phosphorus,
	  magnesium, fluoride, selenium

Comments

Mean nutrient intake should not be used to assess nutrient adequacy

This measure is not appropriate for food energy, given the correlation between
   intake and requirement
This measure is not appropriate for calcium, vitamin D, pantothenic acid, biotin,
   and choline, since they currently do not have an EAR

There currently is no UL for thiamin, riboflavin, vitamin B_{12}, pantothenic acid,
   and biotin, thus no conclusion can be drawn regarding potential risk of
   adverse effects.

Conduct multiple regression analyses of nutrient intakes; compare regression-
   adjusted mean intake for the different subgroups
Regression-adjusted mean nutrient intake should not be used to assess nutrient
   adequacy

Statistical tests of significance can be used to determine if the differences across
   subgroups in percentages less than the EAR are statistically significant
This measure is not appropriate for food energy, given the correlation between
   intake and requirement
This measure is not appropriate for calcium, vitamin D, fluoride, pantothenic
   acid, biotin, and choline, since they currently do not have an EAR

Statistical tests of significance can be used to determine if the differences across
   subgroups in percentages greater than the UL are statistically significant
This measure is not appropriate for nutrients for which a UL has not been set
   (thiamin, riboflavin, vitamin B_{12}, pantothenic acid, and biotin)

centage of the population or group with usual intakes exceeding the UL.

MINIMIZING POTENTIAL ERRORS IN ASSESSING INTAKES

Users of the Dietary Reference Intakes (DRIs) have many opportunities to increase the accuracy of dietary assessments by ensuring that the dietary data are complete, portions are correctly specified, and food composition data are accurate, and by selecting appropriate methodologies and plans for sampling group intakes.

When assessing the dietary adequacy of populations, having accurate information on the distribution of usual (habitual) intakes based on accurate and quantitative food intake information for each individual is necessary. Thus, the use of semi-quantitative food-frequency questionnaires is seldom appropriate for assessing the adequacy of dietary intake of groups.

Physiological measures are helpful when assessing the dietary status of individuals or of groups of people. They can be used to supplement or confirm estimates of inadequacy based on dietary data.

Despite the occurrence of unavoidable errors, it is worthwhile to compare high-quality intake data with accurate requirement data for assessing intakes. At a minimum, such a comparison identifies nutrients likely to be either under- or overconsumed by the individual or the group of interest.

RECOMMENDATIONS FOR RESEARCH TO ENHANCE USE OF THE DRIs

In several parts of this report, only some very general guidelines for applying the Dietary Reference Intakes (DRIs) in dietary assessment are provided. It became clear during development of the report that much research is still needed in this area. By highlighting these areas, it is hoped that there will be a greater chance that research on these topics will be undertaken.

The topics given below are not necessarily in order of priority. Increased knowledge in any of the areas listed would be beneficial in enhancing use of the DRIs for dietary assessment.

Research to Improve Estimates of Nutrient Requirements

Even for nutrients for which an Estimated Average Requirement (EAR) is available, the EARs and Recommended Dietary Allowances (RDAs) are often based on just a few experiments with very small sample sizes. For nutrients with an Adequate Intake (AI) for age groups older than infants, new research and data that allow replacement of the AIs with EARs and RDAs will greatly aid the assessment of nutrient adequacy. In addition, information on the distribution of requirements is needed so that the appropriate method for assessing the prevalence of inadequacy for groups can be determined (EAR cut-point method vs. full probability approach).

Research should be undertaken to allow Tolerable Upper Intake Levels (ULs) to be set for all nutrients and to generate information on ways to identify and conceptualize the risk of exceeding the UL.

Research to Improve the Quality of Dietary Intake Data

The estimation and amelioration of bias (such as under- or over-reporting of food intake) is a relatively unexplored field. Efforts in the management of bias during data analysis are very preliminary and far from satisfactory at present. This is seen as a high priority area waiting for new initiatives and innovative approaches.

Advances in behavioral research to determine why people under-report food intake would allow development of improved dietary data collection tools that would not trigger this behavior. Such information would also help in the derivation of statistical tools to correct the bias associated with this phenomenon.

Better ways to quantify the intake of supplements are needed. A large proportion of the population in the United States and Canada consumes dietary supplements. Using intakes only from food sources in dietary assessment is certain to result in a faulty estimate of nutrient inadequacy, as well as inaccurate estimates of the percentage of the population with intakes above the UL.

Food composition databases will need to be updated to include the forms and units that are specified by the DRIs. Chemical methodology to facilitate analysis of various forms of certain nutrients (e.g., α-tocopherol vs. γ-tocopherol) may be required for comparison to the DRIs.

Research to Improve Statistical Methods for Using DRIs to Assess Intakes of Groups

Methods for developing standard errors for prevalence estimates should be investigated. Some sources of variance (primarily associated with intake data) can currently be quantified but many (such as those associated with requirement estimates) cannot. Without a standard error estimate, it is not possible to determine if an estimated prevalence of X percent is significantly different from zero or if prevalence estimates for two groups of individuals differ significantly from each other or from zero.

Additional research is needed for applications that assess the nutrient intakes of different subgroups of the population. In particular, further research is needed to apply the methods included in this report to estimate differences in the prevalence of inadequacy between subgroups after controlling for other factors that affect nutrient intake.

Ways to assess the performance of methods to estimate prevalence of inadequacy should be investigated. A detailed investigation of the effect of violating assumptions for the EAR cut-point method discussed in this report is a high research priority. This would best be done using well-designed, well-planned, and well-implemented simulation studies. Results of such studies would permit identification of recommendations as to the best approach to be used in assessments for each nutrient and would provide an estimate of the expected bias in prevalence estimates when the conditions for application of the cut-point method are not ideal.

I

Historical Perspective and Background

Part I presents an overview of the report and information on the evolution of dietary reference standards.

Chapter 1 outlines the purpose of this report and provides an introduction to Dietary Reference Intakes (DRIs), a set of four nutrient-based reference values, each of which has special uses.

A discussion of the concept of using dietary reference standards along with the identification of their past uses (specifically the former Recommended Dietary Allowances [RDAs] and Recommended Nutrient Intakes [RNIs]) is detailed in Chapter 2.

1

Introduction and Background

The purpose of this report—one of a series resulting from a comprehensive effort initiated by the Institute of Medicine's Food and Nutrition Board to expand the approach to the development of dietary reference standards—is to assist nutrition and health researchers and other professional users of dietary reference standards in the transition from using the former Recommended Dietary Allowances (RDAs) and Canadian Recommended Nutrient Intakes (RNIs) to using all of the new Dietary Reference Intakes (DRIs) appropriately (a detailed discussion of the origin and framework for development of the DRIs is presented in Appendix A). This report reviews the scientific literature regarding the uses of dietary reference standards and their applications, and provides guidance on the application of DRIs to assess the nutrient intakes of groups and individuals. Application of DRIs in planning diets of groups and individuals will be presented in a subsequent report.

PURPOSE OF THE REPORT

This report focuses on application of the DRIs in *dietary assessment* and is meant as both a "how to" manual and a "why" manual. In this light, specific examples of both appropriate and inappropriate uses of the DRIs in assessing the nutrient adequacy of intakes for groups and for individuals are included. The statistical background that justifies the use of DRIs as described in this report is also included. The detailed statistical approaches for the methods described here have been grouped into appendixes; the text in the main body of

21

the report is precise, but should not require extensive background in statistics to be useful.

An important consideration in the application of the DRIs in both assessment and planning is that a nutrient requirement is defined as the lowest continuing intake level of a nutrient that will maintain a defined level of nutriture in an individual. The criterion of nutritional adequacy on which requirements are based differs among nutrients, and may also differ for a given nutrient depending on the life stage of individuals. The criterion used, the rationale for its selection, and any functional indicators are described in depth in each of the nutrient reports in this series (IOM, 1997, 1998b, 2000). The criterion or criteria chosen for a specific nutrient is for the healthy U.S. and Canadian populations and may not be the most appropriate criterion for other populations. This has important implications for those using the DRIs in assessment or planning. For example, agreement between assessment of dietary intake and assessment of nutritional status cannot be expected if the criterion used to determine the requirement and the criterion used in clinical and biochemical examination for other purposes are not the same.

For the DRIs published at the time this report went to press, the requirement for each nutrient is presented as a single reference intake (amount) for various life stage and gender groups rather than as multiple endpoints. This approach differs from that of the joint World Health Organization and Food and Agriculture Organization Expert Consultation on requirements of vitamin A, iron, folate, and vitamin B_{12} (FAO/WHO, 1988), which recommended both a basal requirement (the amount of nutrient needed to prevent clinically detectable impairment of function) and a normative storage requirement (the amount of nutrient needed to maintain a desirable level in tissues). The single endpoints established for DRIs currently available are more in keeping with a normative storage requirement than a basal requirement.

WHAT ARE DRIs?

Dietary Reference Intakes (DRIs) are relatively new to the field of nutrition. The DRIs are a set of at least four nutrient-based reference values that can be used for planning and assessing diets and for many other purposes. They are meant to replace the former Recommended Dietary Allowances (RDAs) in the United States and Recommended Nutrient Intakes (RNIs) in Canada. The DRIs differ from the former RDAs and RNIs in that (1) where specific data on

safety and efficacy exist, reduction in the risk of chronic degenerative disease—rather than just the absence of signs of deficiency—is
included in the formulation of the recommendation; (2) where data
are adequate, upper levels of intake are established to prevent risk
of adverse effects; and (3) components of food that may not fit the
traditional concept of an essential nutrient but are of possible benefit to health will be reviewed and if sufficient data exist, reference
intakes will be established.

Where adequate information is available, each nutrient will have
a set of DRIs. A nutrient will have either an Estimated Average
Requirement (EAR) and RDA, or an Adequate Intake (AI). When
an EAR for the nutrient cannot be determined (and therefore,
neither can the RDA), then an AI is provided for the nutrient. In
addition, most nutrients will have a Tolerable Upper Intake Level
(UL). Like the former RDAs and RNIs, each type of DRI refers to
the average daily nutrient intake of apparently healthy individuals
over time, although the amount may vary substantially from day to
day without ill effect in most cases.

In developing recommended intakes, emphasis is placed on the
reasons underlying the particular criterion of adequacy used to
establish the requirement for each nutrient. A table of the recommended daily intakes developed using the DRI process, at the time
this report was printed, can be found at the end of this book.

The EAR

The EAR[1] is the median usual intake value that is estimated to
meet the requirement of half the healthy individuals in a life stage
and gender group. At this level of intake, the other half of the
individuals in the specified group would not have their needs met.
The EAR is based on a specific criterion of adequacy, derived from
a careful review of the literature. Reduction of disease risk is considered along with many other health parameters in the selection of
that criterion. The EAR is used to calculate the RDA.

---

[1] It is recognized that the definition of the EAR implies a median as opposed to
a mean or average. The median and average would be the same if the distribution
of requirements followed a symmetrical distribution such as the normal, and would
diverge as a distribution became skewed. Two considerations prompted the choice
of the term EAR: (1) data are rarely adequate to determine the distribution of
requirements, and (2) precedent has been set by other countries that have used
the term EAR for reference values similarly derived (COMA, 1991).

The RDA

The RDA is the average daily dietary intake level that is sufficient to meet the nutrient requirement of nearly all healthy individuals in a particular life stage and gender group. If the distribution of requirements in the group is assumed to be normal, then the RDA is the value that exceeds the requirements of 97 to 98 percent of the individuals in the group (Figure 1-1). Under the assumption of normality, the RDA can be computed from the EAR and the standard deviation of requirements (SD_{REQ}) as follows:

$$RDA = EAR + 2\ SD_{REQ}$$

If the distribution of requirements is normal, 97 to 98 percent of the individuals in the group will have a requirement that is below the RDA. The RDA is intended for use primarily as a goal for usual intake of individuals. Because the RDA is derived directly from the EAR, if data are insufficient to establish an EAR, no RDA can be set.

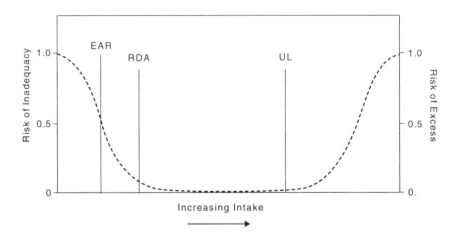

FIGURE 1-1 Dietary reference intakes. This figure shows that the Estimated Average Requirement (EAR) is the intake at which the risk of inadequacy is 0.5 (50 percent) to an individual. The Recommended Dietary Allowance (RDA) is the intake at which the risk of inadequacy is very small—only 0.02 to 0.03 (2 to 3 percent). The Adequate Intake (AI) does not bear a consistent relationship to the EAR or the RDA because it is set without being able to estimate the requirement. At intakes between the RDA and the Tolerable Upper Intake Level (UL), the risks of inadequacy and of excess are both close to 0. At intakes above the UL, the risk of adverse effects increases.

The AI

If sufficient scientific evidence is not available to establish an EAR and set an RDA, an AI is derived instead. The AI is based on experimentally derived intake levels or approximations of observed mean nutrient intakes by a group (or groups) of apparently healthy people who are maintaining a defined nutritional state or criterion of adequacy. Examples of defined nutritional states include normal growth, maintenance of normal levels of nutrients in plasma, and other aspects of nutritional well-being or general health.

The AI would not be consistently related to the EAR and its RDA even if they could be established. For example, for young infants, the AI is usually based on the daily mean nutrient intake supplied by human milk for healthy, full-term infants who are exclusively fed human milk. For adults, the AI may be based on data from a single experiment (e.g., the AI for choline [IOM, 1998b]), based on estimated dietary intakes in apparently healthy population groups (e.g., the AIs for biotin and pantothenic acid [IOM, 1998b]), or result from a review of data from different approaches (e.g., the AI for calcium, based on calcium retention, factorial estimates of requirements, and limited data on bone mineral density and bone mineral content changes in adult women [IOM, 1997]). The AI is expected to exceed the EAR and the RDA for a specified criterion of nutritional adequacy. When an RDA is not available for a nutrient (since there is no EAR), the AI can be used as the goal for an individual's intake. However, as is explained later in this report, the AI has limited uses in assessment.

The issuance of an AI indicates that more research is needed to determine, with some degree of confidence, the mean and distribution of requirements for that specific nutrient. When this research is completed, it should be possible to replace estimates of AIs with EARs and RDAs.

The UL

The UL is the highest level of continuing daily nutrient intake that is likely to pose no risk of adverse health effects in almost all individuals in the specified life stage group (Figure 1-1). As intake increases above the UL, the potential risk of adverse effects increases. The term *tolerable intake* was chosen to avoid implying a possible beneficial effect. Instead, the term is intended to connote a level of intake with a high probability of being tolerated biologically. The UL is not intended to be a recommended level of intake. Unless specifically identified in the nutrient reports (e.g., for folate in the prevention of neural tube defects [IOM, 1998b]), there is no currently established benefit to healthy individuals associated with ingestion of nutrients in amounts exceeding the RDA or AI.

The UL is based on an evaluation conducted using the methodology for risk assessment of the adverse effects of nutrients (IOM, 1998a). The need to establish ULs grew out of the increasingly common practice of fortification of foods with nutrients and the increased use of dietary supplements. For some nutrients, data may not be sufficient for developing a UL. This indicates the need for caution in consuming high intakes and should not be interpreted as meaning that high intakes pose no risk of adverse effects.

General Properties of DRIs

Unless otherwise stated, all values given for EARs, RDAs, AIs, and ULs represent the total quantity of the nutrient or food component to be supplied by foods (including nutrients added to foods) and by nutrients ingested as supplements. These values are also based on usual or continuing intakes. The DRIs apply to the apparently healthy population. RDAs and AIs are not expected to replete individuals who are already malnourished, nor are they intended to be adequate for those who may have increased requirements because of certain disease states. Appropriate goals for intake should be provided to those with greatly increased nutrient requirements. Although the RDA or AI may serve as the basis for such guidance, qualified medical and nutrition personnel should make necessary adaptations for specific situations.

Comparison of the AI with the RDA

In general, both values are intended to cover the needs of nearly all members of a life stage group. For both RDAs and AIs, values for children and adolescents may be extrapolated from adult values if no other usable data are available. However, there is much less certainty about an AI value in comparison to an RDA value.

The RDA is based on specific knowledge of the requirement and assumptions about its distribution and is set to meet the requirements of almost all (97 to 98 percent) of the population. In contrast, the AI is an experimentally derived or observed mean intake that appears to maintain a specific criterion of adequacy in a group of apparently healthy people. Therefore, by definition, the RDA incorporates only the estimated variability in requirements, whereas the AI, if based on observed mean intakes, incorporates the variability of both requirements and intake. The AI represents an informed judgment about what seems to be an adequate intake for an individual based on available information, whereas the RDA is a more data-based and statistically relevant estimate of the required level of intake for almost all individuals. For this reason, AIs must be used more carefully than RDAs.

Criteria of Adequacy

In the derivation of the EAR or AI, close attention has been paid to determining the most appropriate criteria of adequacy. A key question is, Adequate for what? In many cases a continuum of benefits may be ascribed to various levels of intake of the same nutrient. Each EAR and AI is described in terms of the selected criterion or, in some cases, criteria. For example, the EAR, and thus the RDA, for folate for women of childbearing age is based on a combination of biochemical indicators or criteria. A separate recommendation is made for women capable of becoming pregnant to reduce the risk of a neural tube defect in the offspring if pregnancy occurs. There are many possible and equally legitimate criteria of adequacy. The criteria are discussed in each nutrient report as part of the rationale for the DRIs developed (IOM, 1997, 1998b, 2000).

Uncertainty in Requirement Estimations

The task of setting both median requirements (EARs) and ULs for apparently healthy persons of all ages and both genders in various physiological states is ambitious. Ideally, data from the target population on intakes at various levels and the functional effects of these intakes would be available. In reality the information base is often limited, and its reliability varies from nutrient to nutrient. These limitations are discussed in detail in each of the nutrient reports (IOM, 1997, 1998b, 2000). Users of these reports should recognize that the DRIs are estimates based on available data, and that even when an EAR, RDA, and a UL for a nutrient are provided for a life stage and gender group, there is considerable uncertainty about these values. The DRIs will continue to evolve as better information becomes available. When interpreting the results of assessments of individuals or groups, it is appropriate to consider possible limitations in the information base that was used to generate the relevant DRIs.

ORGANIZATION OF THE REPORT

This report is organized to take the user step-by-step through methodology for using the Dietary Reference Intakes (DRIs) to assess the adequacy of nutrient intakes. An overview of the concept of using dietary reference standards along with the identification of their past uses (specifically the former Recommended Dietary Allowances [RDAs] and Recommended Nutrient Intakes [RNIs]) is presented in Chapter 2.

Chapter 3 describes how DRIs can be used for assessing the apparent nutrient adequacy of individuals, and includes a discussion of obtaining and interpreting information on individual intakes and the effect of the large within-person variation. Examples of specific applications are also provided.

Chapter 4 provides the statistical basis for the use of the Estimated Average Requirement (EAR) in assessing nutrient adequacy of groups. The chapter begins with a basic discussion of the concept of assessing the prevalence of inadequate nutrient intakes and then develops the statistical approaches for estimating this prevalence. Assumptions required for the use of the statistical models are discussed, as is the need for adjusting intake distributions.

In Chapter 5, the focus is on group-level assessment of nutrient adequacy using the Adequate Intake (AI). Chapter 6 provides guidance on the extent to which the Tolerable Upper Intake Level (UL) can be used to estimate the prevalence of potential risk for adverse effects in groups.

Specific guidance with examples on appropriate applications of the DRIs for group assessment purposes is provided in Chapter 7—the methodological approaches described in Chapters 4, 5, and 6 are applied to some of the specific uses of dietary reference standards reported in Chapter 2. Three specific applications are presented and discussed.

A brief description of limitations in the measurement of intakes and requirements, and the importance of accurate sampling techniques are highlighted in Chapter 8. Chapter 9 provides recommendations for research needed to improve and refine nutrient assessments.

2

Current Uses of
Dietary Reference Standards

This chapter begins with a brief discussion of the history of dietary recommendations for nutrients in the United States and Canada. This discussion includes a conceptual framework that both describes two main general uses of the dietary reference standards and is the basis for organizing the remainder of this report. The next section catalogues the current uses of dietary reference standards on the basis of information provided by the U.S. and Canadian federal agencies involved in health and nutrition policy.

CHANGES OVER TIME

Since the publication of the first Recommended Dietary Allowances (RDAs) for the United States in 1941 and Daily Recommended Nutrient Intakes (DRNIs) for Canada in 1938 (now shortened to RNIs), applications of quantitative recommended intakes have expanded both in scope and diversity. Uses range from their original objective to serve as a goal for good nutrition to such diverse uses as food planning and procurement, design and evaluation of food assistance programs, development of nutrition education materials, food labeling, food fortification, and dietary research.

Primary Applications

In 1941, the Food and Nutrition Board first proposed the RDAs "to serve as a goal for good nutrition and as a 'yardstick' by which to measure progress toward that goal..." (NRC, 1941, p. 1). Even today,

29

many of the specific uses and applications of dietary reference standards fall into the two general categories defined implicitly in 1941—diet planning and diet assessment. Diet planning applications involve using dietary reference standards to develop recommendations for what intakes should be (i.e., as a goal for good nutrition). Diet assessment applications involve determining the probable adequacy or inadequacy of observed intakes (i.e., a yardstick by which to measure progress). These two general applications of dietary reference standards are interrelated.

The first Canadian dietary standards—DRNIs—were issued by the Canadian Council on Nutrition (1938) and stated that the standards were to be used as the basis for evaluation of observed diets. It was not clear whether group diets (group mean intakes) or individual diets were intended.

The 1990 version of the RNIs and 1989 RDAs did not differ in the described derivations of the recommended intakes but differences remain about how intended uses are described, resulting in some confusion for the users of both reports. The joint U.S. and Canadian development of the new Dietary Reference Intakes (DRIs) should resolve this confusion.

Conceptual Framework

Figure 2-1 illustrates a conceptual framework adapted from one first developed by Beaton (1994) which can be applied to the uses of dietary reference standards. As shown in this figure, knowledge about distributions of requirements and intakes feeds into the two general applications of diet planning and assessment. Within each of these general categories, the applications differ according to whether they are for an individual or for population groups.

The simplicity of this conceptual framework belies the complexity in using and interpreting DRIs to plan and assess diets. In the past, both planning and assessment applications relied primarily on the former RDAs or RNIs because these were the only quantitative nutrient reference standards widely available. The concepts underlying the former RDAs often were not well understood and thus some applications of the former RDAs for both assessment and planning were not appropriate (IOM, 1994). For the three newly introduced dietary reference intakes—the Estimated Average Requirement (EAR), Adequate Intake (AI), and Tolerable Upper Intake Level (UL)—guidance is needed to differentiate which should be used in various applications in diet assessment and planning. As discussed in the next section, the wide range of uses for dietary

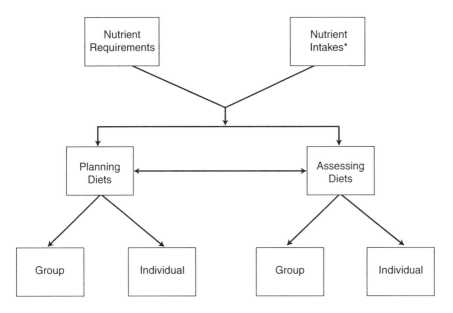

FIGURE 2-1 Conceptual framework—uses of dietary standards. *Food plus supplements.
SOURCE: Adapted from Beaton (1994).

reference standards represents both the importance of developing scientifically based standards and the need to assist the user in understanding fully how each DRI should be used and interpreted.

USES OF THE FORMER RDAs AND RNIs

Users of dietary reference standards include those who plan meals for individuals and groups; individual consumers who decide what foods to eat and how much; the food industry which produces, voluntarily fortifies, and markets foods; federal, state, and local government agencies that design, operate, and evaluate food and nutrition assistance programs; scientific and regulatory bodies that formulate standards and regulations to ensure marketed foods are safe and appropriately advertised; and nutrition and health professionals who educate, counsel, evaluate, and monitor public health.

Table 2-1 and the following text includes the major applications for which the Recommended Dietary Allowances (RDAs) and Rec-

TABLE 2-1 Reported Uses of Dietary Reference Standards[a]

General Use of Dietary Reference Standards	Assessment (A) or Planning (P)
Evaluation of Dietary Data	
Assess nutrient intake of individuals	A
Assess nutrient intakes of groups	A
Nutrition Education and Guides for Food Selection	
Evaluate an individual's diet as a basis for recommending specific changes in food patterns and nutrient needs	A
Evaluate nutrient intakes of groups as a basis for nutrition education sessions	A
Provide guidance to individuals and groups on how to obtain a nutritious diet	P
Develop food guides and dietary guidelines	P

Specific Identified Uses of Dietary Reference Standards

Compare an individual's nutrient intake with Recommended Dietary Allowances (RDA) or Recommended Nutrient Intakes (RNI)

Compare nutrient intakes with RDA or RNI to estimate the percentage of the population at risk of inadequate intake based on percent of RDA or RNI

Compare nutrient intakes—mean, median, and distributions of intake—with RDA or RNI for population subgroups to determine the size and type of populations considered to be at risk of inadequate intake

Compare nutrient intakes with RDA or RNI to assess variations over time in the percentage of the population at risk of inadequate intake based on prevalence below RDA or RNI

Monitor the potential of the food supply to meet the nutritional needs of the population, examine trends, and evaluate changes over time in diets

Compare an individual's nutrient intake with dietary reference standards and identify changes in food consumption patterns that might reduce the risk of inadequate intake

Compare nutrient intakes of population subgroups with dietary reference standards and identify changes in food consumption patterns that might reduce the risk of inadequate intake; identify foods that are important contributors of nutrients

Counsel individuals and educate groups on selecting foods to meet required nutritional standards

Use in developing and revising the U.S. Department of Agriculture's Dietary Guidelines for Americans and the Food Guide Pyramid, and Canada's Food Guide to Healthy Eating, which provide information on types and amounts of foods that meet nutritional requirements

continued

TABLE 2-1 Continued

General Use of Dietary Reference Standards	Assessment (A) or Planning (P)
Food and Nutrition Assistance Programs	
Develop plans for feeding groups to meet nutritional standards and for food budgeting and purchasing	P
Develop food packages for program benefits	A, P
Evaluate meals and foods offered by programs	A
Design food and nutrition assistance programs	A
Evaluate the dietary effects of food and nutrition assistance programs	A
Determine eligibility for the Special Supplemental Nutrition Program for Women, Infants, and Children (WIC)	A
Military Food and Nutrition Planning and Policy	
Nutrition research	A
Food procurement and meal planning	P

Specific Identified Uses of Dietary Reference Standards

Use dietary reference standards and typical food-purchasing patterns to define four official U.S. Department of Agriculture food plans: (1) the Thrifty Food Plan, used as the basis for the Food Stamp Program; (2) and (3) the moderate and liberal food plans, used as the basis for military food allowances; and (4) the low-cost food plan, used for financial planning in bankruptcy and other similar court cases

Design meal patterns that provide a specified percentage of the dietary reference standards for the National School Lunch Program, the School Breakfast Program, the Child and Adult Care Feeding Program, and the Summer Food Service Program

Use as a basis for evaluating and modifying nutrient content of food packages for the Special Supplemental Nutrition Program for Women, Infants, and Children (WIC), the Food Distribution Program on Indian Reservations, and the Commodity Supplemental Food Program

Compare nutrients offered at meals—means, medians, and distributions—with program regulations

Compare nutrient intakes—mean, median, and distributions of intake—with dietary reference standards to identify population subgroups for possible intervention with food assistance, fortification, and education

Compare nutrient intakes—mean, median, and distributions of intake—with dietary reference standards, by program participation; estimate program effects and estimate the percentage, by program participation status, at risk of inadequate intake

Compare individual nutrient intake with dietary reference standards to assess whether an individual is at nutritional risk on the basis of an inadequate diet

Determine whether dietary reference standards need to be adjusted for field conditions (peacetime, peacetime overseas, conflict, war)

Compare nutrient intakes with dietary reference standards to evaluate the ability of the military meal planning to meet nutritional standards

Use dietary reference standards as a basis for planning meals for the military and use of fortified foods, supplements, special food products

continued

TABLE 2-1 Continued

General Use of Dietary Reference Standards	Assessment (A) or Planning (P)
Military rations and deployment policies	P
Nutrition education	P
Institutional Dietary Assessment and Planning	A, P
Assessment of Disease Risk	A
Food Labels and Nutritional Marketing	P
Clinical Dietetics	
Develop therapeutic diet manual	P
Counsel patients requiring modified diets and plan modified diets	P
Assess patient intakes to determine if nutritional supplementation is needed	A
Food Fortification and Development of New or Modified Food Products	A, P
Food Safety Considerations	A

a This table is based on a survey of federal agencies in the United States and Canada and appropriateness.

Specific Identified Uses of Dietary Reference Standards

Use dietary reference standards to set military rations
Determine military rations based on adjusted dietary reference standards for field
   conditions—Nutritional Standards for Operational Rations

Develop nutrition education material for military personnel to counsel them how
   to meet required nutritional standards and how to avoid overconsumption

Use dietary reference standards to assess the adequacy of, and as a basis for,
   planning meals in institutional settings such as hospitals, dormitories, prisons,
   and nursing homes

Use epidemiological analyses relating nutrient intakes to health and nutritional
   status

Use dietary reference standards as reference points for deriving nutrient
   reference standards for food labels
Use dietary reference standards to communicate information on the nutrient
   content of foods

Use dietary reference standards as a basis for modifying menu plans for patient
   groups requiring therapeutic diets

Use dietary reference standards as benchmark for modifying the diets of
   individual patients requiring therapeutic diets

Use dietary reference standards as a basis for assessing the individual's observed
   intake

Compare nutrient intakes of population subgroups with dietary reference
   standards to determine which nutrients are inadequately consumed;
   fortification may be mandated by government or voluntary by the food industry
Use by industry as a guide for developing new or modified food products

Compare nutrient intakes with dietary reference standards to identify the size
   and type of populations at risk from use of particular foods and food products;
   identify extreme and unusual patterns of intakes of foods, food ingredients, or
   food additives; and determine the need to enact or modify regulations

onducted in 1998. It summarizes reported uses and does not represent any judgment about ommended Nutrient Intakes (RNIs) have been used in the past, although there may be other uses that are not identified here.

Evaluation of Dietary Data

Dietary reference standards have been used to evaluate dietary intake data for individuals, frequently in conjunction with biochemical, clinical, or anthropometric data. They can also be used to evaluate intake data for groups of individuals. Possible uses in evaluating groups include: estimating the percentage of the population at risk of inadequate or excessive intake; identifying subgroups at risk of inadequate or excessive intake; examining changes over time in the percentage of the population and of population subgroups at risk of inadequate or excessive intake; monitoring the potential of the food supply to meet the nutritional needs of the population; and examining trends and changes in food consumption over time.

Nutrition Education and Guides for Food Selection

Nutrient standards (specifically, the former RDAs and RNIs) have long been the foundation for discussing nutrient needs, for comparing the nutritional value of foods, and for counseling individuals and groups on how to meet nutritional requirements as part of nutrition education (Sims, 1996). Dietary assessment also provides information for nutrition education efforts and guides food selection. By linking findings from dietary assessment with foods consumed, it is possible to identify foods that are important contributors of nutrients, specify food consumption patterns that might reduce the probability of dietary inadequacy, and educate individuals and groups about appropriate foods and food consumption patterns. The difficulty encountered in applying dietary reference standards for this purpose is in translating quantitative nutrient recommendations into food-based information for dietary planning. Food guides, such as the U.S. Department of Agriculture's (USDA) Food Guide Pyramid and Health Canada's Food Guide to Healthy Eating, attempt to do just this. These guides group foods according to their nutrient contributions and provide recommendations for selecting the types and amounts of foods that provide the recommended intakes for most nutrients (Welsh et al., 1992). It may be difficult, however, to develop food guides which meet the RDAs and AIs for all nutrients, and consideration of the Tolerable Upper Intake Level (UL) in developing or modifying food guides will provide an additional challenge.

Food and Nutrition Assistance Programs

Quantitative nutrient recommendations have been the cornerstone of food and nutrition assistance programs. In the United States, the RDAs have been used: (1) as the basis for specified meal patterns in child nutrition programs and other institutional feeding programs; (2) as the nutritional goals of the Thrifty Food Plan, a low-cost food plan that determines benefit levels for the Food Stamp Program; (3) in development of food packages and benefits for various targeted nutrition programs such as the Special Supplemental Nutrition Program for Women, Infants, and Children (WIC); and (4) in assessment of compliance with USDA nutrition program regulations. There are few government-operated nutrition assistance programs in Canada and thus, no equivalent reported uses of the RNIs.

Similarly, dietary reference standards—typically the former RDAs and RNIs—have been used as guidelines for planning meals by incorporation into regulations for feeding groups (e.g., school children or elderly adults) and for making food purchasing and budgeting decisions.

In general, when the former RDAs were used to plan diets, the goals were set such that a certain percentage of the RDA was achieved over a period of a week or longer. The challenge for those who have used the former RDAs and RNIs for planning meals and designing food and nutrition program benefits will be how to incorporate the new reference standards of Estimated Average Requirements (EARs), RDAs, Adequate Intakes (AIs), and ULs to enhance and improve the nutritional dimension of diet planning.

Military Food and Nutrition Planning and Policy

The U.S. Department of Defense uses dietary reference standards for dietary assessment, food procurement and meal planning, setting nutrient levels of military rations for deployment, and developing nutrition education materials for military personnel. Nutrient standards are used by the military to plan menus and meals for garrison feeding and to assess whether provision of fortified foods, nutrient supplements, or special food products are needed in operational conditions. For example, in the past the military adapted the former RDAs to reflect variations in physical activity or stress or to emphasize performance enhancement (rather than to prevent deficiencies) (AR 40-25, 1985).

Institutional Dietary Assessment and Planning

People who are fed in institutional settings vary in demographic and life stage characteristics (e.g., day care centers vs. long-term care facilities), health status, expected duration of residence (e.g., a school vs. a correctional facility), and proportion of total dietary intake obtained from institutional food services (e.g., a single congregate meal program vs. a nursing home). Institutions also vary in their characteristics, such as whether clients consume food in the facility or at another location (e.g., congregate vs. home-delivered meals), availability and degree of food choice offered to clients or residents, food budgets, ownership (public or private), legal requirements pertaining to food or nutrient composition of the diet served, and the means used to assess and monitor whether nutrient needs of clients are met.

In general, institutions that cater to individuals at high nutritional risk and those that provide clients with most or all of their food on a long-term basis have a particular need to plan diets or menus that allow individuals to consume nutrients at levels comparable to nutrient recommendations.

The former RDAs and RNIs have been widely used as the basis for menu planning for groups and as goals to achieve in interventions aimed at improving the nutritional quality of individual meals or overall diets. They have also been used as benchmarks against which intakes are assessed (e.g., the proportion of residents achieving the RDA or RNI). Specific categories of DRIs may be more appropriate for some of these purposes.

Assessment of Disease Risk

Much of the knowledge of the relationships between nutrients and specific diseases comes from clinical and epidemiological studies of diet and disease in diverse human populations. Thus, epidemiological research is used to identify possible relationships between specific dietary components and observed disease patterns. In turn, the dietary reference standards can be used to assess intakes and exposure to nutrients in the study of a nutrient's relationship to risk of dietary deficiency diseases, chronic diseases, or adverse effects resulting from excessive intake or exposure.

Food Labels and Nutritional Marketing

Food labeling is a highly visible application of the use of quantitative nutrient standards. As of 2000, food labels in both the U.S. and Canada still use values based on older standards (1983 Recommended Daily Nutrient Intakes in Canada and 1968 RDAs in the United States). In addition to providing consumers with information on the nutrient content of food products, the nutrient standards serve as a basis for nutrient content claims and health claims. For example, in the United States, if a food label contains a claim that the food is a good source of a vitamin, that food must contain at least 10 percent of the Daily Value (DV) for that vitamin in the serving portion usually consumed. The DV is based on the Reference Daily Intake, which was usually based on the highest RDA for adolescents or adults as established in the 1968 RDAs (NRC, 1968). To make a health claim with regard to lowering the risk of a chronic disease, a food must meet specific regulatory guidelines with respect to the required content of the nutrient for which the health claim is made. The food industry often uses messages on food labels to communicate and market the nutritional benefits of food products.

Clinical Dietetics

RDAs and RNIs have also been used as the basis for planning menus for groups of hospital patients, as a reference point for modifying diets of patients, and as a guide for the formulation of oral nutritional supplements or of complete enteral and parenteral feeding solutions. The use of quantitative nutrient standards for developing therapeutic diets and counseling patients requires caution since in the past, and now with the DRIs, these standards were established to meet the needs of almost all apparently *healthy* individuals. Those with therapeutic needs may not have their needs met, or they may have specific clinical conditions that would be worsened by consuming a nutrient at the recommended level. In developing therapeutic diets for patients with a specific disease, the usual procedure is first to use recommended intakes for nutrients that are not affected by the disease. For other nutrients, estimates are based on the best evidence of needs during illness. These assumptions are usually specified in the diet manuals of hospitals and professional associations.

Food Fortification and Development of New or Modified
Food Products

Public health professionals and the food industry also use the results from dietary assessment to identify nutrients that appear to be inadequate in groups evaluated and then to consider either fortifying foods or developing new foods to assist in meeting nutrient needs. Fortification can be of significant benefit when a large segment of the population has usual intakes of a nutrient below the dietary standard and nutrition education efforts have been ineffective. Food fortification in the United States may be mandatory, such as in the folate, iron, and selected B vitamin fortification of cereal grains, or voluntary, as in the addition of a large array of vitamins in ready-to-eat cereals. The effects of fortification on intake distributions depend on the choice of food fortified.

Food Safety Considerations

Dietary assessment provides information for people concerned with the food safety considerations associated with the prevalence of very high intakes of nutrients. Information on how to apply the UL should be helpful here.

LOOKING AHEAD: APPLYING THE DRIs

The introduction of the Dietary Reference Intakes (DRIs), especially the Estimated Average Requirement (EAR) and Tolerable Upper Intake Level (UL), provides better tools for many of the uses described here and presented in Table 2-1. This report presents how specific DRIs should be used for dietary assessment. While some examples of application in the assessment of individuals and of groups are provided, not all of the uses described above are specifically addressed. A subsequent report will discuss using specific DRIs in planning.

II

Application of DRIs for Individual Diet Assessment

In Part II, the focus is on how to assess nutrient adequacy of individuals using the Dietary Reference Intakes (DRIs).

Chapter 3 demonstrates how to compare an individual's intake to the appropriate DRI of a nutrient to decide, with a predetermined level of confidence, whether an individual's intake of a nutrient is adequate or excessive. A discussion on obtaining and interpreting information on individual intakes and the effect of the large within-person variation is included and examples of specific applications are provided.

3

Using Dietary Reference Intakes for Nutrient Assessment of Individuals

This chapter provides a statistical approach to those wishing to quantitatively assess an individual's diet relative to the Dietary Reference Intakes (DRIs). The information presented in this chapter should be kept in context. Those who actually conduct individual assessments typically have access to a variety of information sources, including: (1) types of foods in the diet and information on usual dietary patterns; (2) lifestyle practices (e.g., smoking, alcohol consumption, exercise patterns); (3) anthropometric data; (4) clinical diagnosis (e.g., diabetes, cholesteremia, hypertension, cardiovascular disease); and (5) information on nutrient intakes from analysis of food records or recalls. Although the information presented in this chapter focuses on nutrient intake data, it should always be considered in combination with other information in dietary assessment of individuals.

Throughout the chapter, the fact that an individual's observed mean intake over a few days may not be an accurate estimate of that individual's usual intake is emphasized. When comparing mean observed intake to a DRI, it is important to take into account the day-to-day variability in intake. In addition, an individual's requirement of a nutrient is almost always unknown, and this uncertainty must also be accounted for in individual assessment. Specifically, this chapter demonstrates how to compare an individual's intake to the appropriate DRI of a nutrient to decide, with a predetermined level of confidence, whether an individual's intake of a nutrient is adequate or excessive.

The statistical approaches proposed in this chapter are not applicable to all nutrients because they assume normal distributions of daily intakes and requirements. A different methodology needs to be developed for nutrients for which the requirement distribution in the population is skewed (such as the iron requirements of menstruating women) or for which the distribution of daily intakes is skewed (as in the case of vitamin A, vitamin B_{12}, vitamin C, vitamin E, and perhaps several others). Until these new methods are available, individual assessment for these nutrients should continue to place emphasis on the types of information mentioned above for a qualitative assessment.

INTRODUCTION

When an Estimated Average Requirement (EAR) for a nutrient is available, it is possible to make a quantitative assessment of the adequacy of the individual's usual intake of the nutrient. When an Adequate Intake (AI) is all that is available, it is still possible to determine whether the individual's usual intake is above the AI with a predetermined level of confidence. No conclusions can be drawn, however, when usual intake is below the AI. In this chapter, guidance is provided on how to determine whether an individual's usual intake of a nutrient exceeds the Tolerable Upper Intake Level (UL), suggesting that the usual intake is excessive. Note that use of the Recommended Dietary Allowance (RDA) is *not recommended for individual assessment.*

Whether one is interested in assessing the adequacy of the individual's usual intake or in deciding whether usual intake exceeds the UL, the relevant information must include both the observed mean intake and the standard deviation (*SD*) of daily intakes for the individual. In the next section it is emphasized that usual intake is unobservable in practice, but for the purposes of assessment, it suffices to observe the individual's daily intake over a few days and to have a reliable estimate of the *SD* of daily intake.

PROPOSED NEW METHOD FOR INDIVIDUAL ASSESSMENT

Is an individual's diet meeting nutrient needs? This question is fundamental to individual nutrition counseling and education. Answering this question is not an exact science, and the answer is considerably less precise than might be anticipated, especially because of the *appearance* of accuracy in computer printouts providing nutrient analysis of dietary intake data.

The Dietary Reference Intakes (DRIs) can be used to assess the apparent adequacy of an individual's intake to maintain the state of nutriture used to define a requirement. However, DRIs can neither provide precise quantitative assessments of the adequacy of diets of individuals nor be used to exactly assess nutritional status. Diet software programs based on the DRIs cannot do so either.

Assessing dietary adequacy by comparing an individual's intake and requirement for a nutrient is problematic for two reasons: first, the *individual's requirement* for a given nutrient must be known, and second, the *individual's usual intake* of the nutrient must be known. As described in Chapter 1, *requirement* is defined as the lowest continuing intake level of a nutrient that will maintain a defined level of nutriture in an individual for a given criterion of nutritional adequacy. *Usual intake* is defined as the individual's average intake over a long period of time. As is evident from these definitions, determining an individual's exact requirement would involve a controlled clinical setting in which the individual would be fed graded levels of a particular nutrient over a period of time, while undergoing numerous physiological and biochemical measurements. Determining usual intake requires a prohibitively large number of accurate diet records or recalls assessed using accurate food composition information (see Chapter 8 for further discussion of the importance of accurate intake and food composition data). Because neither type of information is usually available, it is simply not possible to *exactly* determine whether an individual's diet meets his or her individual requirement.

For some nutrients, however, it is possible to approximately assess whether an individual's nutrient intake meets his or her requirement. The remainder of this chapter and Appendix B provide specific guidance to help professionals assess individual dietary intake data relative to the DRIs. To do so, it is necessary to obtain information on an individual's usual intake, choose the appropriate reference standard, and then interpret the intake data.

Whenever possible, the assessment of apparent dietary adequacy should consider biological parameters such as anthropometry (e.g., weight for height), biochemical indices (e.g., serum albumin, blood urea nitrogen, creatinine, retinol binding protein, hemoglobin), diagnoses (e.g., renal disease, malabsorption), clinical status, and other factors as well as diet. Dietary adequacy should be assessed and diet plans formulated based on the totality of the evidence, not on dietary intake data alone.

Obtain Information on the Individual's Usual Intake

The first step in individual assessment is to obtain the most accurate information possible on total dietary intake (food and supplements), recognizing that this is always a challenge because of the documented high incidence of underreporting (Johnson et al., 1998; Lichtman et al., 1992; Mertz et al., 1991), and the large day-to-day variation in intake (Beaton et al., 1979, 1983; Gibson, 1990; Sempos et al., 1985; Tarasuk and Beaton, 1991b, 1992; Van Staveren et al., 1982). Intake on one or even several days may give very inaccurate estimates of usual intake, especially if the individual's food choices vary greatly from one day to the next, which is a common occurrence. Following are some issues to consider when determining the magnitude of day-to-day variation:

- Factors that affect day-to-day variation in nutrient intake include:
  — variety versus monotony in an individual's food choices (Basiotis et al., 1987; Sempos et al., 1985; Tarasuk and Beaton, 1991b, 1992)
  — day of the week (Beaton et al., 1979; Tarasuk and Beaton, 1992; Van Staveren et al., 1982)
  — season
  — holidays and special occasions
  — appetite (which may be related to changes in physical activity, the menstrual cycle, etc. [Barr et al., 1995; Tarasuk and Beaton, 1991a])
- The number of days needed to estimate usual intake also varies according to the desired precision of the estimate (see examples in Box 3-1). Obtaining an estimate within ± 10 percent of the usual

---

BOX 3-1 The Number of Days Needed to Estimate Usual Intake Varies with the Specific Nutrient and the Desired Precision

Consider trying to estimate an individual's usual intake of niacin and vitamin C. In a study of 13 men over 1 year, it was estimated that determining mean niacin intake within ± 10 percent of their true usual intake required 53 days of intake data, whereas 249 days of intake data were needed to estimate usual vitamin C intake with the same precision. In a study of 16 adult women over 1 year, an average of 222 days of intake data was needed to estimate their vitamin C intake within ± 10 percent of true usual intake, while an estimate within ± 20 percent of true usual intake required only 55 days (Basiotis et al., 1987).

intake requires more days of intake data than obtaining an estimate within ± 20 percent of the usual intake (Basiotis et al., 1987).

• Special attention must be given to nutrients that are highly concentrated in a few foods that are consumed only occasionally (see vitamin A example in Box 3-2). It takes fewer days to estimate usual intake of nutrients found in lower concentrations in many foods, especially if those foods are dietary staples (Gibson et al., 1985).

Nutrient intakes of individuals are estimated using instruments (e.g., diet records, recalls, diet histories, or food-frequency questionnaires) that are seldom capable of capturing long-term usual intake. With careful attention to technique (i.e., instruments that capture total nutrient intake such as food records and dietary recalls), and access to complete food composition databases, these instruments may provide an accurate reflection of the individual's intake during a specified time period (e.g., a 3-day record). Suggestions for improving the accuracy of dietary intake data collection are discussed further in Chapter 8. See Box 8-1 for a list of issues to consider when estimating dietary intake.

However, because of day-to-day variation in intake (within-person variation), this *observed* intake is probably not the same as long-term *usual* intake. In all likelihood, an individual's observed intake during one 3-day period will differ from observed intake in another 3-day period, and both 3-day observed intakes will differ from true usual intake. There is also error due to within-person variation with instruments such as food-frequency questionnaires, and some authors have estimated this error to be similar to that seen with 3-day records and recalls (Beaton, 1991; Liu, 1988). Diet histories may have less

---

BOX 3-2 The Challenge of Estimating Usual Vitamin A Intake

Consider trying to estimate an individual's usual intake of vitamin A. On four consecutive days, a person might consume 600, 750, 250, and 400 retinol equivalents (RE). Does the average of these four values (500 RE) represent usual intake over a longer time, such as 1 year? In most cases it would not, because vitamin A intake is often extremely variable. The intake on the next day might be 100 or 4,000 RE, changing the estimated usual intake to 420 or to 1,200 RE, respectively. Very different conclusions would be drawn about the likely adequacy of this individual's diet from these different estimates, but would any of these estimates be correct? Probably not. Estimating usual vitamin A intake requires months, if not years, of records.

error from within-person variation, but the size of this error has not been quantified.

It is clear that estimating an individual's usual intake for a nutrient from the individual's observed intake alone may lead to an under- or overestimation of that individual's usual intake of the nutrient. However, it is still possible to evaluate the potential error if something is known about the magnitude of the within-person variation in intakes for that nutrient. The individual's observed mean intake is the best estimate available of the individual's usual intake of the nutrient. A pooled estimate of the within-person variability in intakes has been computed for a number of nutrients from nationwide food consumption surveys (see Appendix Tables B-2 through B-5). The magnitude of the day-to-day variation in intakes of a nutrient will indicate whether the observed mean intake calculated from a few daily records or recalls is a more or less precise estimator of the individual's usual intake of that nutrient. The observed mean intake and the pooled estimate of day-to-day variability in intakes will be used subsequently to guide individual dietary assessments.

Choose the Appropriate Reference Standard

The second step in individual assessment is to choose the appropriate DRI to use as a reference standard. In assessing the apparent adequacy of an individual's intake, interest is in whether the individual's nutrient requirement is met. Unfortunately, information on an individual's requirement is seldom, if ever, available. Therefore, the best estimate for an individual's unobservable requirement is the Estimated Average Requirement (EAR), defined as the median requirement of a nutrient for a given life stage and gender group. Obviously there is variation in requirements among individuals, and assumptions have been made about the shape of the requirement distribution. A coefficient of variation (*CV*) (standard deviation of the requirement divided by the mean requirement × 100) of 10 percent has been assumed for most of the nutrients for which EARs have been established (IOM, 1997, 1998b, 2000). If requirements are normally distributed, a *CV* of 10 percent means that about 95 percent of individuals would have requirements between 80 and 120 percent of the EAR (± 2 standard deviations). With a *CV* of 15 percent, as has been estimated for niacin (IOM, 1998b), the corresponding range would be between 70 and 130 percent of the EAR. For some nutrients the *CV* of the requirement distribution may be even higher, and for other nutrients (e.g., iron requirements of menstruating women) the requirement distribution is known to be skewed rather than normal. *For nutrients with skewed requirement distributions, the approach to assess individual intakes proposed in this chapter is not appropriate.*

The larger the *CV* (and thus the standard deviation), the larger the range of possible values for an individual's requirement for that nutrient, and the greater the uncertainty about what the individual's requirement for that nutrient might be. Even in the hypothetical case in which the individual's usual nutrient intake is known, uncertainty remains about whether the usual intake is adequate, because that individual's requirement is not known.

Recommended Dietary Allowances (RDAs) have been established as a target or goal for intake by an individual, and it can be assumed that individuals whose *usual* intakes are above the RDA are likely to be meeting their individual requirements and thus have adequate intakes. However, the converse is not true. For this reason the RDA is not a useful reference standard for assessing an individual's intake. Intakes below the RDA cannot be assumed to indicate that an individual's intake is inadequate. The RDA, by definition, exceeds the actual requirements of all but 2 to 3 percent of the population, so many of those with usual intakes below the RDA may be meeting their individual requirements. The likelihood of nutrient inadequacy, however, increases as the usual intake falls further below the RDA.

As discussed in the previous section, however, usual intakes are unobservable in practice. Thus, one is limited to comparing the observed mean intake to the DRIs in order to assess adequacy. Subsequently in this chapter it will be demonstrated that due to the typically high day-to-day variability in intakes for most nutrients, one may not be able to conclude that an individual's usual intake is adequate even if the observed mean intake is larger than the RDA. Thus, *comparing an individual's observed mean intake to the RDA is not recommended as a means for determining nutrient adequacy for the individual.*

If an Adequate Intake (AI) rather than an EAR was set for a nutrient (e.g., calcium, vitamin D), it may be used in a more limited way as described in the next section.

Interpret Individual Dietary Intake Data

The third step in individual assessment is to assess the data to answer the question, On the basis of an individual's observed intake over a small number of days, is that individual's *usual* intake of the nutrient adequate and at low risk of adverse effects?

Using the Estimated Average Requirement

As described earlier in this chapter, trying to compare an individual's intake to his or her requirement for a nutrient is difficult for two main reasons: (1) one needs to know an individual's *requirement;* and (2) one needs to know an individual's long-term *usual intake* of the nutrient. Neither the individual's requirement nor the usual intake of an individual is known.

Appendix B presents in detail a proposed approach, summarized below, to address this issue, recognizing that nutrient requirement and usual intake are not observable for a given individual. This approach is based on the following assumptions:

• The EAR is the best estimate of an individual's requirement.
• There is person-to-person variation in requirements. The standard deviation of the requirement is an indicator of how much the individual's requirement for a nutrient can deviate from the median requirement (EAR) in the population.
• Mean observed intake of an individual is the best estimate of an individual's usual intake.
• There is day-to-day variation in intake for an individual. The within-person standard deviation of intakes is an indicator of how much observed intake may deviate from usual intake.

Inferences about the adequacy of an individual's diet can be made by looking at the difference between observed intake and the median requirement. That is, D is the difference between the mean observed intake for an individual ($\bar{y}$) and the median requirement (EAR, called r for simplicity) for the life stage and gender group to which the individual belongs,

$$D = \bar{y} - r.$$

If the difference D is large and positive, that is, if observed intake is much greater than the median requirement, then it is likely that an individual's intake is adequate. Conversely, if the difference D is large and negative, that is, observed intake is much less than the median requirement, then it is likely that an individual's intake is not adequate. In between, there is considerable uncertainty about the adequacy of the individual's intake.

The obvious question then, concerns how large D would have to be before it could be concluded with some degree of assurance that the individual's unobservable usual intake exceeds the individual's unobservable actual requirement. To answer this question, it is necessary to know the standard deviation of D (SD_D). The SD_D depends on the number of days of intake available for the individual, the standard deviation of the requirement (estimated as 10 to 15 percent of the EAR for most nutrients), and the within-person standard deviation of intake. The latter can be estimated from large surveys of similar groups of people (such as the Continuing Survey of Food Intakes by Individuals [CSFII] data presented in Appendix Tables B-2 through B-5). Once D and SD_D have been estimated, the probability that intake is above (or below) the requirement can be determined by examining the ratio of D to SD_D.

To illustrate this approach, suppose a 40-year-old woman had a magnesium intake of 320 mg/day, based on three days of dietary records. The question is whether this observed mean intake of 320 mg/day of magnesium over three days indicates that her usual magnesium intake is adequate. The following information is used in conducting this assessment:

• The EAR for magnesium for women 31 to 50 years of age is 265 mg/day, with an SD of requirement of 26.5 mg/day.
• The day-to-day SD in magnesium intake for women this age is 85.9 mg/day based on data from the CSFII (see Appendix Table B-2).

The following steps can now be used to determine whether an intake of 320 mg/day is likely to be adequate for this woman.

1. Calculate the difference D between intake and the EAR as $320 - 265 = 55$ mg.
2. Use the formula for the SD_D[1] and determine that the SD_D is 56 mg. The value of SD_D is computed as follows: (a) from Appendix Table B-2, the pooled SD of daily intake for magnesium in women aged 19 to 50 years is 86 mg/day, and therefore the variance of daily intake is the square of the SD or 7,379 mg; (b) divide 7,379 by the number of days of observed intake data (3) to obtain 2,460;

---

[1] $SD_D = \sqrt{\left(V_r + V_{within} / n\right)}$, where V_r denotes the *variance* of the distribution of requirements in the group, and V_{within} denotes the average variance in day-to-day intakes of the nutrient. Both variances are computed as the square of the corresponding standard deviations. Intuitively, as the number n of intake days available on the individual increases, the variance of the observed mean intake should decrease (i.e., the accuracy of the estimate for y increases). Thus, the dividing V_{within} by n when computing the standard deviation of the difference D.

(c) add this to the square of the SD of requirements ([26.5 mg/day]^2 = 702 mg/day), resulting in a value of 3,162; and (d) the SD_D is then obtained as the square root of 3,162, which is 56.

3. Therefore, D (55) divided by SD_D (56) is just slightly less than 1. As shown in Appendix Table B-1, a value of about 1 implies an 85 percent probability of correctly concluding that this intake is adequate for a woman in this age category. (Details and further explanation are given in Appendix B.)

It is important to note that this woman's intake was exactly equal to the RDA of 320 mg/day, yet since there are only three days of dietary records, there is only 85 percent confidence that this intake is adequate. Only if true long-term intake had been measured for this woman (which is seldom feasible) could there be 97.5 percent confidence that intake at the RDA is adequate. With only three days of dietary recalls, it would be necessary for her magnesium intake to be 377 mg/day (which is well above the RDA) in order to have 97.5 percent confidence that intake was adequate (see Table 3-1).

Note that the SD of daily intake for the woman is not estimated from her own 3-day records. Instead, the estimated SD of daily intake of magnesium obtained from the CSFII is used. This estimate is a pooled (across all sampled individuals of the same life stage and gender group) SD of daily intake.

Why not use the woman's three days of intake records to estimate her SD of daily intake? As discussed earlier in this chapter, daily intakes may vary considerably from one day to the next. Unless the three days of intake recorded for the woman represent her entire range of intakes of magnesium, the SD that is estimated from her own records is likely to be severely biased. Thus, it is recommended that the pooled SD of daily intake obtained from the CSFII (or from other similar large-scale dietary surveys) be used for individual assessment. This has one serious drawback, however, as it is well known that the SD of daily intake also varies from individual to individual. In particular, it has been suggested that the within-person SD of intake is larger in those individuals with higher consumption of the nutrient (Tarasuk and Beaton, 1991a). Nusser et al. (1996) suggested that for some nutrients the association between mean intake and SD of intake for the individual is approximately linear. At this time, however, no extensive studies have been conducted to allow reliable estimation of the within-person SD of intakes from the individual's intake records. Therefore, even though the pooled SD obtained from CSFII (or other large-scale dietary surveys)

TABLE 3-1 Illustration of Observed Mean Intakes of Magnesium That Would Be Necessary to Have 85 Percent or 97.5 Percent Confidence That Usual Intake Is Greater Than the Requirement for a Woman 40 Years of Age

	Using SD of Intake from CSFII[a]		Assuming the SD is 25 Percent Larger		Assuming the SD is 50 Percent Larger	
	mg	% RDA[b]	mg	% RDA	mg	% RDA
Magnesium EAR[c]	265		265		265	
SD of requirement	26.5		26.5		26.5	
Magnesium RDA	320		320		320	
Assumed SD of intake[d]	86		107		129	
Observed mean intake with 85% confidence of adequacy of usual intake						
1 d of intake	355	111	376	117	397	124
3 d of intake	321	100	332	104	344	107
7 d of intake	307	96	313	98	320	100
Observed mean intake with 97.5% confidence of adequacy of usual intake						
1 d of intake	445	139	486	152	528	165
3 d of intake	377	118	400	125	423	132
7 d of intake	349	109	362	113	376	117

NOTE: Observed mean intake with *xx* percent confidence of adequacy = observed mean intake necessary to have approximately *xx* percent confidence that the woman's intake is greater than her requirement.

[a] SD = standard deviation; CSFII = Continuing Survey of Food Intake by Individuals.

[b] RDA = Recommended Dietary Allowance for women 31 through 50 years of age.

[c] EAR = Estimated Average Requirement for women 31 through 50 years of age.

[d] SD of magnesium intake for women 19 through 50 years of age taken from CSFII (Appendix Table B-2).

is not the best estimate of the individual's *SD* of daily intake, the Subcommittee still recommends its use in individual assessment.

Table 3-1 expands this example to further illustrate the effect of day-to-day variation on the evaluation of magnesium intake for a woman in the 31–50 years age group.

• For a given confidence level, the number of days of intake data affects the level of nutrient intake judged to be adequate. Based on the *SD* in intake of 85.9 mg/day for an individual (again using the information in Appendix Table B-2), observed intake would need to be 445 mg/day (139 percent of the RDA) to have a 97.5 percent confidence that intake was adequate with only one day of observed intake. However, a mean observed intake of only 349 mg/day (109 percent of the RDA) would be needed with 7 days of observed intake.

• For a given confidence level, the larger the *SD* of daily intake, the greater the intake level needed for intake to be assessed as adequate. If the *SD* of magnesium intake were 25 percent larger, then intake would need to be 486 mg/day (152 percent of the RDA) to have a 97.5 percent confidence of adequacy with one day of observed intake, and 362 mg/day (113 percent of the RDA) with 7 days. If the *SD* were 50 percent larger, then the intakes would need to be still higher to have 97.5 percent confidence of adequacy.

To simplify this approach for nutrition professionals, institutions, and agencies may wish to establish levels of intake that they consider adequate for a given nutrient. For the example shown here, a level of 377 mg/day might be chosen as the level of adequacy of magnesium intake for women 31 to 50 years of age, by an institution that typically collects three days of dietary data for its patients, and wanted a high level of confidence (97.5 percent) that intake was adequate.

To summarize, despite the fact that neither individual requirement nor usual individual intake is available for dietary assessments of individuals, some inferences about individual adequacy can be made by looking at the difference between observed intake and the median requirement. Shortcomings of this approach are described in Appendix B. For example, the approach cannot be used when observed daily intakes are not normally (or symmetrically) distributed around the individual's usual intake. An indication that the within-person intake distribution is not normal (or symmetrical) is the size of the within-person standard deviation in intake relative to the mean intake. When the *SD* of daily intake is high enough so that the *CV* of daily intake is larger than approximately 60 to 70 percent, then the approach proposed here is not appropriate. Appendix Tables B-2 and B-3 indicate that for vitamin A, carotenoids, vitamin C, and vitamin E, among others, the *CV* of daily intake is very large, above 70 percent. For those nutrients, it would be incorrect to apply the method described in this section to assess adequacy of an individual's diet. At this time, no alternative can be offered, as much research is needed in this area.

It is also possible to calculate observed nutrient intake levels with an 85 or 97.5 percent confidence of *inadequacy*. Intakes with a high probability of inadequacy are below the EAR. For confidence (at

97.5 percent) that an observed intake is below an individual's requirement, it is necessary to have either a large number of days of intake or for the intake to be substantially below the EAR. Taking magnesium for women 19 through 50 years of age as an example, with 7 days of observed intake, an intake of about 180 mg/day (compared with the EAR of 265 mg/day) would have a high probability (97.5 percent) of being below an individual's requirement. However, it is often the case that a nutrition professional wants to have a high level of confidence when concluding that intakes are *adequate* but will find a much lower level of confidence acceptable when concluding that intake is *inadequate*. For example, even if the probability of inadequacy was only 50 percent, most professionals would urge a client to try to increase intake of that nutrient. One would want to be much more certain before concluding that a client's intake was adequate and that no action to improve intake was needed.

Thus, for practical purposes, many users of the DRIs may find it useful to consider that observed intakes below the EAR very likely need to be improved (because the probability of adequacy is 50 percent or less), and those between the EAR and the RDA probably need to be improved (because the probability of adequacy is less than 97.5 percent). Only if intakes have been observed for a large number of days and are at or above the RDA, or observed intakes for fewer days are well above the RDA, should one have a high level of confidence that the intake is adequate. It is hoped that computer software will be developed that will compute these probabilities (as described in Appendix B), thus offering more objective alternatives when individual intakes are evaluated.

In summary, for nutrients for which an EAR has been established, it is possible to assess the adequacy of an individual's usual intake for a nutrient. The approach described above takes into account the uncertainty about the true value of the individual's usual intake, and also the uncertainty about the individual's requirement for the nutrient. The method cannot be employed when the distribution of requirements for the nutrient is skewed (as in the case of iron requirements for menstruating women), or when the distribution of daily intakes for an individual is not normal (as is the case with nutrients for which the *CV* of intake has been calculated to be above 60 to 70 percent, see Appendix Tables B-2 through B-5). There are three additional sources of potentially large error when using this approach to assessing an individual's intake:

• The assumed 10 percent *CV* estimate applied to many nutrients to date (IOM, 1997, 1998b, 2000) may not be a reliable estimator of the *SD* of requirement. Since the *SD* of requirement is an important component of the SD_D, an inaccurate value for the *SD* of requirement will result in an inaccurate value for SD_D and hence the ratio of D/SD_D.

• The *SD* of daily intake for the individual is considerably larger (or smaller) than the pooled *SD* of daily intake obtained from CSFII (or from the National Health and Nutrition Examination Survey).

• The individual's intake is underreported, so that the mean observed intake is a biased estimator of the individual's usual intake.

The described approach should not be used in isolation from other information available to nutrition professionals. Most professionals combine the nutrient intake data with other sources of information such as food guides and answers to questions about whether intake was typical or atypical.

This statistical approach to individual assessment is based on quantitative dietary records and recalls, where the method for deriving the error term (the within-person standard deviation of intakes) is known and easy to apply. Many researchers and health professionals use other methods of estimating usual intakes, such as food frequencies or diet histories, or a combination of various methods. With alternative assessment methodologies, the overall objective of the assessment remains the same—to determine whether usual intake by the individual exceeds the individual's requirement—and professionals must rely on estimates of both usual intake and requirement. The important consideration is that different methodologies for determining dietary intake have different sources and magnitudes of random error in estimating usual intake—the equivalent of the within-person standard deviation of intake discussed above—and may not provide adequate quantitative estimates of total nutrient intake over the period of observation. Additional discussion of dietary intake measurement instruments is provided in Chapter 8. However, a detailed discussion of these methods is beyond the scope of this report, and users will need to turn to other sources to find estimates of the error associated with alternative methods for estimating usual intake.

Using the AI

If an AI must be used to interpret dietary intake data because an EAR has not been set, the process described above cannot be used in the same way. Before discussing a statistical approach to individual assessment for nutrients with an AI, it is critical to emphasize the difference between these two DRIs. The EAR represents the median nutrient requirement of a given life stage and gender group, and by definition, an intake at the level of the EAR will be inadequate for half the group. In contrast, the AI represents an intake (not a requirement) that is likely to exceed the actual (but unknown) requirements of almost all healthy individuals in a life stage and gender group. In this respect it is analogous to the RDA; however, because of the nature of the data used to establish AIs, they may often be higher than the RDA would be if appropriate data were available to calculate one.

The approach discussed previously to assess nutrient adequacy compares an individual's observed intake to the EAR, and considers variability in both intakes and requirements when determining how confident one can be in concluding that an individual's intake is adequate. In other words, intakes are compared to the *median requirement*. In the case of the AI, however, intakes are compared to an *intake* value *in excess* of the median requirement, perhaps by a very large margin. Thus, when intakes are compared to the AI, all one can truly conclude is whether intake is above the AI or not. Although an intake that is significantly above the AI is certainly adequate, intakes below the AI are also likely to be adequate for a considerable proportion of individuals. Thus, great caution must be exercised when interpreting intakes relative to AIs.

What conclusions can be drawn about individual intakes for nutrients with AIs?

First, if an individual's **usual** *intake exceeds the AI, it can be concluded that their diet was almost certainly adequate. However, if their* **usual** *intake falls below the AI, no quantitative estimate can be provided of the likelihood of nutrient inadequacy.*

Risk of inadequacy increases at some point below the AI. If the usual nutrient intake from all sources was zero, the risk of inadequacy would be virtually 100 percent. However, because the point where risk increases cannot be determined, quantitative estimates of risk cannot be made.

Even if the observed intake is above the AI, it should not be assumed that usual intake is above the AI unless a large number of days of intake data were collected. As discussed in the previous section on the EAR, it is difficult to collect dietary intake data that truly reflect usual intake.

Can an approach similar to the one described earlier be developed to assess whether an individual's usual intake is above the AI? The answer to this question is yes, but with some reservations. When the EAR is not available, there is no information about the distribution of requirements in the population. One can, nonetheless, test whether an individual's usual intake exceeds the AI, and if so, conclude that the individual's usual intake is likely to be adequate. A test similar to the one presented in the preceding section incorporates the day-to-day variability in intakes in order to determine whether *usual* intake for the individual is above the AI.

As an example, consider a nutrient for which the AI has been determined to be 500 units/day, the individual being assessed is a woman 40 years of age, with three dietary recalls, and a mean observed intake of 560 units/day. The *SD* of daily intake for this nutrient is 50 units (as might be listed in Appendix Table B-2). To decide whether the woman's usual intake is above the AI, one would follow these steps:

1. Compute the difference between the woman's observed mean intake and the AI. In this example, the difference is $560 - 500 = 60$ units.

2. Divide the difference by the *SD* of daily intake over the square root of the number of days of intake available for the woman. In this example, $50/\sqrt{3} = 29$, and $60/29 = 2.07$.

3. Compare 2.07 to the tabulated values shown in Appendix Table B-6, and find the confidence level with which one could conclude that the woman's usual intake was above the AI. In this case, 2.07 corresponds to a high confidence level of about 98 percent.

For this woman, it can be confidently concluded that her usual intake of the nutrient is at or above the AI and thus adequate. This procedure, therefore, can be used to determine whether usual intake is larger than the AI given the observed intake for a few days.

Given an observed mean intake for the individual the confidence with which one can determine usual intake to be above the AI depends on: (1) the number of days of observed intake available for the individual, and (2) the *SD* of daily intake for the nutrient. An example using calcium intake is provided in Table 3-2. In this example, observed mean intake of calcium relative to the AI for calcium is assessed for a woman 40 years of age. Different numbers of daily

TABLE 3-2 Illustration of the Computations Necessary to Test Whether Usual Intake Is Above the Adequate Intake (AI) for Different Numbers of Days of Observed Intake for a Woman 40 Years of Age

	Using SD from CSFII[a]	If SD is 25 Percent Larger	If SD is 50 Percent Larger
Mean intake	1,200 mg	1,200 mg	1,200 mg
SD of intake[b]	325 mg	406 mg	488 mg
AI for calcium[c]	1,000 mg	1,000 mg	1,000 mg
z-Values = (mean intake − AI)/(SD/square root [n])			
1 d of intake	0.61	0.49	0.41
3 d of intake	1.07	0.85	0.71
7 d of intake	1.69	1.30	1.08
Percentage confidence that the woman's usual intake exceeds the AI[d]			
1 d of intake	73	69	66
3 d of intake	86	80	76
7 d of intake	95	90	86

NOTE: The confidence with which one can conclude that usual intake is greater than the AI decreases when the number of days of daily intake records for the individual decreases, or when the SD of daily intake increases.

[a] SD = standard deviation; CSFII = Continuing Survey of Food Intake by Individuals.

[b] SD of calcium intake for women 19 through 50 years of age taken from CSFII (Appendix Table B-2).

[c] Adequate Intake for women 31 through 50 years of age.

[d] Confidence values were taken from a standard z-table (Snedecor and Cochran, 1980). The z-table is used because the SD of daily intake is assumed to be known (e.g., from CSFII), and is not computed from the woman's daily observations.

intake records and different *SDs* of daily intake for calcium were assumed. For each case, the confidence with which one would conclude that her usual intake is above the AI was calculated and is shown in the table.

If one can conclude that in fact usual intake appears to be larger than the AI with desired accuracy, then there is considerable assurance that the individual's intake is adequate. However, if the test does not result in the conclusion that usual intake is larger than the AI with the desired precision, then it cannot be inferred that intake is inadequate.

As discussed earlier, this approach is not appropriate when daily intakes for an individual are not approximately normally distributed.

TABLE 3-3 Qualitative Interpretation of Intakes Relative to the Adequate Intake (AI)

Intake Relative to AI	Suggested Qualitative Interpretation
Greater than or equal to the AI	Mean intake is likely adequate if observed over a large number of days
Less than the AI	Adequacy of intake cannot be determined

Any nutrient for which the *CV* of daily intakes exceeds about 60 to 70 percent has a skewed daily intake distribution and therefore the test described here cannot be applied. In those cases, a qualitative interpretation of the observed mean intake may be all that is available. Table 3-3 gives some guidance on to how to interpret mean observed intake relative to the AI qualitatively.

Using the UL

If a nutrient has a UL, that value can be used to assess the likelihood that an individual may be at risk of adverse affects from high intake of the nutrient. Doing so requires a good understanding of the definition of the UL and the type of intake (e.g., foods, fortified foods, and/or supplements) that should be considered during the assessment.

The UL is a level of chronic daily nutrient intake that is likely to pose no risk of adverse health effects for almost all individuals in the general population, including sensitive individuals. For many nutrients, the UL reflects intake from all sources, including food, water, nutrient supplements, and pharmacological agents. However, in some cases the UL applies only to intakes from fortified foods and supplements or intakes from supplements only. As stated previously (see Chapter 1), ULs do not represent *optimal* or *desirable* intakes but instead are intakes that should generally not be exceeded by healthy individuals. An occasional intake above the UL by a small margin is not a reason for major concern. However, because it is not possible to know who is most susceptible to adverse effects of intakes above the UL, such intakes should be avoided.

What if an individual has an intake above the UL on a chronic basis? For example, what if a person's magnesium intake from a nonprescribed antacid is 500 mg per day and the UL for magnesium (based on supplemental intake only) is 350 mg?

The most prudent advice in this situation would be to recommend that the individual reduce intake to below the UL. In this example, choosing a different type of antacid might be appropriate.

The consequences associated with nutrient excess—severity and reversibility of the adverse effect—vary for different nutrients. Moreover, little is known about nutrient-nutrient interactions at high doses. Without good evidence for an expected benefit, or unless under the supervision of a physician, there is no justification for intake above the UL.

If an individual decides to take a supplement for nontherapeutic purposes, should a supplement that contains the UL of a nutrient be selected?

No, supplements should not be chosen on this basis.

Use of a supplement containing the UL for a nutrient, when combined with intakes from foods, would place the individual at potential risk of adverse effects. Accordingly, a supplement which contains nutrients at levels below, or approximating the RDA or AI would be a more appropriate choice.

A test similar to the one described in the preceding section for the AI can be implemented to decide whether usual intake is below the UL given the observed mean intake. The test is constructed in exactly the same manner, but now the UL is subtracted from the mean observed intake for the individual. Again, this test cannot be used for nutrients with a large *CV* of daily intake such as vitamin A, vitamin B_{12}, vitamin C, and vitamin E (see Appendix Tables B-2 and B-3).

An example similar to the one presented in Table 3-2 is presented in Table 3-4. In the example, again the assessment is for a woman who is 40 years old. This woman has a normal activity pattern, energy intake not exceeding 2,500 kcal/day, and a mean phosphorous intake of 3.8 g (see IOM [1998b] for discussion of high phos-

TABLE 3-4 Illustration of the Computations Necessary to Test Whether an Individual's Usual Intake of Phosphorus Is Below the Tolerable Upper Intake Level (UL) for Different Numbers of Days of Observed Intake for a Woman 40 Years of Age

	Using SD from CSFII[a]	If SD is 25 Percent Larger	If SD is 50 Percent Larger
Mean intake	3.8 g	3.8 g	3.8 g
SD of intake[b]	0.4 g	0.5 g	0.6 g
UL for phosphorus[c]	4.0 g	4.0 g	4.0 g
z-Values = (mean intake – UL)/(SD/square root [n])			
1 d of intake	–0.49	–0.39	–0.32
3 d of intake	–0.84	–0.68	–0.56
7 d of intake	–1.29	–1.03	–0.85
Percentage confidence that the woman's usual intake is below the UL [d]			
1 d of intake	69	65	63
3 d of intake	80	75	71
7 d of intake	90	85	80

NOTE: The confidence with which one can conclude that usual intake is below the UL decreases when the number of days of daily intake records for the individual decreases or when the SD of daily intakes increases.

[a] SD = standard deviation; CSFII = Continuing Survey of Food Intake by Individuals.
[b] SD of phosphorus intake for women 19 through 50 years of age taken from CSFII (Appendix Table B-2).
[c] Tolerable Upper Intake Level for women 31 through 50 years of age.
[d] Confidence values were taken from a standard z-table (Snedecor and Cochran, 1980). The z-table is used because the SD of daily intake is assumed to be known (e.g., from CSFII), and is not computed from the woman's daily observations.

phorous intakes associated with high energy expenditure). The UL for phosphorus has been determined to be 4.0 g/day, and the SD of phosphorous intake, from CSFII, is 0.41 g. Given that her observed mean intake is below the UL, can we conclude with desired assurance that her *usual* intake of phosphorus is below the UL and that she is not at potential risk of adverse health effects? Again, situations are shown with 1, 3, and 7 days of intake data.

From the example in Table 3-4, it can be seen that even when *observed mean intake* is less than the UL, sometimes it cannot be concluded with desired accuracy that *usual intake* is also below the UL. When only one day of intake data is available for the individual, one would have only between 63 and 69 percent (depending on the SD of daily intake) confidence in concluding that her intake of 3.8 g reflects a usual intake below the UL. In this example, only the 7 days of intake data provide levels of confidence of 85 to 90 percent for concluding that this woman's usual intake is below the UL given her observed mean intake.

Since this test would be conducted only in cases where the observed mean intake for the individual is high enough to suggest a problem, the *SD* of daily intake as calculated in CSFII or the National Health and Nutrition Examination Survey may underestimate the individual's true *SD* of daily intake. This is because there is some evidence that the *SD* of daily intake increases as the mean intake increases (Nusser et al., 1996). Using a *SD* of daily intake that is too small may lead to the conclusion that usual intake is below the UL when in reality it is not (at a given level of assurance).

As described previously, this test can be performed when daily intakes can be assumed to approximate a normal distribution. An indication that daily intakes are not normally distributed is a high *CV* of intake. From Appendix Tables B-2 through B-5, it can be seen that for several nutrients the *CV* of daily intake is above 60 to 70 percent. In those cases, this test approach is not recommended, and one should make a qualitative assessment of the individual's intake. Table 3-5 presents qualitative interpretations of an individual's intake in relation to the UL. The impact of within-person variation at high intake levels (e.g., levels approaching the UL) has not been studied extensively.

When using the proposed method it is important to note that the pooled estimates of the within-person standard deviation of intakes in Tables B-2 to B-5 are based on data on nutrients from food only, not food plus supplements. This suggests the need for caution in using these estimates in assessing individual intakes relative to the UL. For some nutrients, ULs are defined on the basis of total intake (food plus supplements), and the estimates of the within-person

TABLE 3-5 Qualitative Interpretation of Intakes Relative to the Tolerable Upper Intake Level (UL)

Intake relative to the UL	Suggested Qualitative Interpretation
Greater than or equal to the UL	Potential risk of adverse effects if observed over a large number of days
Less than the UL	Intake is likely safe if observed over a large number of days

standard deviation of intakes based on food alone may not be the same as those based on food plus supplements. For other nutrients, ULs refer only to nutrient intake from food fortificants, supplements, and pharmacological products. In these cases, the proposed methods are even less reliable, as currently there are no estimates of the within-person standard deviation of intakes from supplement use alone.

APPLICATIONS

The following examples show how the Dietary Reference Intakes (DRIs) might be used as part of an assessment of an individual's diet. Note that information other than intake relative to the DRIs is also considered, and in many instances may provide data that are more useful in the assessment than are the nutrient intakes.

Application 1. Assessing the Diet of an Older Individual in an Assisted Living Setting

Background and Data

Mr. G is a 78-year-old man who lives in an assisted-living institution where he eats most of his meals in the dining room. He does not currently take supplements. By observing what he eats, it is possible to obtain direct estimates of his dietary intake, rather than rely on his reports alone, and this is done for several days. Anthropometric data (weight changes), physical activity level, and other information on his health status are available.

Question

The nutritionist who is a consultant to the assisted living facility wants to determine whether Mr. G's food intake is sufficient to meet his nutrient needs.

Assessment

Because it is difficult to determine energy balance, even from several days of intake, the nutritionist determines whether Mr. G is maintaining weight. This is a much more direct method of assessing the adequacy of his energy intake than estimating his caloric intake. In addition to such non-dietary evaluations, the nutritionist obtains an indication of the adequacy of his intake of other nutrients by comparing them to the appropriate DRIs. The assessments that might be made are shown in Table 3-6 for several nutrients from Mr. G's dietary record analysis.

Application 2: Assessing the Diet of a Young Woman Planning a Pregnancy

Background

Ms. T, who is a health-conscious 30-year-old woman, consults a nutritionist in private practice. Before her visit, she keeps a 7-day record of her food and supplement intake, which has been analyzed using a computer program.

Question

Before she becomes pregnant, Ms. T wants to know whether her diet is optimal.

Assessment

With the caveat that 7 days is not long enough to provide accurate information on her usual nutrient intake, her mean observed intake can be evaluated relative to the DRIs. For nutrients with an Estimated Average Requirement (EAR), the nutritionist should calculate the confidence of adequacy using the algorithms described in Appendix B and summarized in this chapter. For nutrients with an Adequate Intake (AI), her intake was adequate if it was likely to exceed the AI (as concluded from the test described in this chapter), whereas no conclusive assessment can be made if her intake was below the AI. Finally, if her intake was not below the Tolerable Upper Intake Level (UL) (as concluded from the test described in this chapter), one would conclude that her usual intake is excessive and she is potentially at risk of adverse effects. This assessment is not appropriate for nutrients with highly skewed requirement distributions (e.g., iron) or large coefficients of variation (CVs) of intake (e.g., vitamin A, vitamin B_{12}, vitamin C, and vitamin E).

Note that data on nutrient intake in relation to the DRIs are only one component of the assessment, and would be interpreted in conjunction with other types of information before counseling was offered. For example, additional information could include: her recent weight history (as an indicator of the likely adequacy of her

TABLE 3-6 Example of Assessing Dietary Adequacy of an Individual

	Thiamin (mg)	Riboflavin (mg)	Folate (µg)[a]	Calcium (mg)	Phosphorus (mg)	Vitamin D (µg)
Mr. G's Mean Intake[b]	1.3	1.1	200	600[c]	1,000	3
RDA[d]	1.2	1.3	400		700	
EAR[e]	1.0	1.1	320		580	
D = Intake − EAR	0.3	0.0	−120		420	
SD Requirement[f]	0.1	0.11	32		58	
SD within[g]	0.69	0.81	150	339	408	
SD of Difference (D)[h]	0.28	0.33	65.1		165	
D/SD_D	1.07	0.0	−1.6		2.5	
AI[i]				1,200		15
Intake − AI				−600		−12
$\dfrac{(\text{Intake} - \text{AI})^c}{(SD_{\text{within}}/\sqrt{7})}$						
Assessment (confidence of adequacy)[j]	About 85%	About 50%	About 5%	No assessment[k]	Over 98%	No assessment[k]
Assessment (qualitative)	Likely to be adequate	Intake should be improved	Intake should be improved		Very likely to be adequate	

[a] Folate is based on µg of folate rather than Dietary Folate Equivalents for this example.

[b] Average of 7 days of intake.

[c] If Mr. G's mean calcium intake had been 1,300 mg instead of 600, one could determine whether intake was adequate after calculating the z-statistic $(1,300 - 1,200)/128$, where 128 is obtained as $339/7$ days. In this case, the resulting z-statistic would have been 0.78, and one would be unable, at any reasonable level of assurance, to conclude that Mr. G's calcium intake is adequate.

[d] RDA = Recommended Dietary Allowance.

[e] EAR = Estimated Average Requirement.

[f] Estimated as EAR × CV.

[g] See Appendix Table B-2.

[h] The standard deviation (SD) of the difference $D = \sqrt{\left(SD_{within}^{2}/7 + SD \text{ of requirement}^{2}\right)}$.

[i] AI = Adequate Intake.

[j] Estimated using the algorithms described in Appendix B; see the Appendix for details of these calculations.

[k] One should use clinical judgment to obtain additional information if intake appears to be extremely low relative to the AI.

energy balance); other information about her diet (to determine how typical her intake was during the 7-day period); whether Ms. T was consuming fortified foods or supplements containing 400 µg of folate (as recommended for women capable of becoming pregnant), a recommendation distinct from the Recommended Dietary Allowance (RDA) and intended to minimize the risk of neural tube defects; and additional information about her lifestyle (e.g., physical activity, use of alcohol).

SUMMARY

The Dietary Reference Intakes (DRIs) can be used in assessment of the apparent adequacy or excess of an individual's dietary intake. Such an assessment requires using the individual's observed mean intake as an estimate of long-term usual intake and using the Estimated Average Requirement (EAR) of the appropriate life stage and gender group as an estimate of the individual's requirement.

For nutrients with an EAR and Recommended Dietary Allowance (RDA), the individual's observed intake in conjunction with measures of variability of intakes and requirements can be used to assess the *likelihood of inadequacy*. For nutrients with an Adequate Intake (AI), the *z*-test described above for the AI can be applied to determine if usual intakes are at or above the AI and can thus be assessed as adequate. For nutrients with a Tolerable Upper Intake Level (UL), the method described above for the UL can be used to determine with a given degree of confidence whether an individual's usual intake is truly below the UL, and therefore is not at risk of adverse health effects.

Remember that in all cases, the individual assessments should be interpreted cautiously, in combination with other types of information.

III

Application of DRIs for Group Diet Assessment

The focus of Part III is on applying the appropriate DRIs for dietary assessment of groups.

Chapter 4 provides the statistical basis for the use of the Estimated Average Requirement (EAR) in assessing nutrient adequacy of groups. The chapter begins with a basic discussion of the concept of assessing the prevalence of inadequate nutrient intakes and then develops the statistical approaches for estimating this prevalence. Assumptions required for the use of the statistical approaches are discussed, as is the need for adjusting intake distributions.

Using the Adequate Intake (AI) for group-level assessment of nutrient adequacy is discussed in Chapter 5. Guidance on the extent to which the Tolerable Upper Intake Level (UL) can be used to estimate the prevalence of risk of adverse effects in groups is provided in Chapter 6.

Specific guidance with examples on appropriate applications of the DRIs for group assessment purposes is provided in Chapter 7. In this chapter, the methodological approaches described in Chapters 4, 5, and 6 are applied to some of the specific uses of dietary reference standards reported in Chapter 2. Three specific applications are presented and discussed.

4

Using the Estimated Average Requirement for Nutrient Assessment of Groups

This chapter describes the use of Estimated Average Requirements (EARs) for assessing the nutrient intakes of groups. It begins with a basic discussion of how to assess conceptually the prevalence of inadequate nutrient intakes and then develops statistical approaches for estimating this prevalence. For some nutrients (those with Adequate Intakes [AIs] rather than EARs such as calcium, vitamin D, fluoride, pantothenic acid, biotin, and choline), the amount and quality of data currently available for both nutrient intakes and requirements may not be sufficient to apply these statistical models in their entirety for purposes of research and policy. Moreover, in addition to assessing nutrient intakes, assessment of health and nutritional status of groups or individuals must include biochemical, clinical, and anthropometric data.

INTRODUCTION

Individuals in a group vary both in the average amounts of a nutrient they consume and in their requirements for the nutrient.

To accurately determine the proportion of a group that has a usual intake of a nutrient less than the requirement, information on both usual intakes and nutrient requirements for each individual in the group is needed. With this information, assessing how many individuals have intakes that do not meet their individual requirements is straightforward. They can just be counted. That is, determine whether each person's usual intake is below his or her requirement, and then count the number of people in the group who do not meet their requirement.

What proportion of individuals in a group has a usual intake of a nutrient that is less than the requirement for that nutrient?

This is one of the most basic questions that can be asked about nutrient intakes, and is critically important from a public health perspective. Clearly, the implications would differ if 30 versus 3 percent of individuals in the population had usual intakes that were inadequate to meet estimated needs. Presented in this chapter is an abbreviated description of a statistical approach to estimating the prevalence of inadequate intakes—the probability approach and a shortcut to the probability approach referred to as the EAR cut-point method. Both of these require the use of the EAR.

Consider a purely hypothetical example of a group comprised of 24 individuals, whose intakes of and requirements for a nutrient are known. The data for these individuals are plotted in Figure 4-1.

In this figure, the 45° line represents the points at which intake equals requirement. The individual labeled "A" in the plot has an intake of the nutrient of 7 units and a requirement for the nutrient of 11 units. Points that fall below (or to the right of) the 45° line are for individuals whose usual intakes are greater than their requirements, whereas points above (or to the left of) the line (the shaded area) are for individuals whose usual intakes are less than their requirements. Six individuals have inadequate intakes, corresponding to the six points above the line. Thus, for this group, the prevalence of inadequate intakes is (6/24) × 100, or 25 percent.

A second example illustrates the same approach with a larger sample. Figure 4-2 shows hypothetical intakes and requirements for a nutrient in a group of 3,000 people. Both the requirement distribution and the intake distribution are assumed to be normal, and not correlated. That is, people who have high requirements do not have a tendency to consume more and thus have greater intakes. The average requirement for the nutrient is 1,200 units and the standard deviation of the requirement is 180 units. The mean of the usual intakes of 3,000 people is 1,600 units and the standard deviation for intake for this group is 450 units. Note that the average usual intake (1,600) is greater than the average requirement (1,200) and that there is more variability (spread) in intakes than there is in requirements. This is the usual situation for most nutrient intakes and requirement distributions.

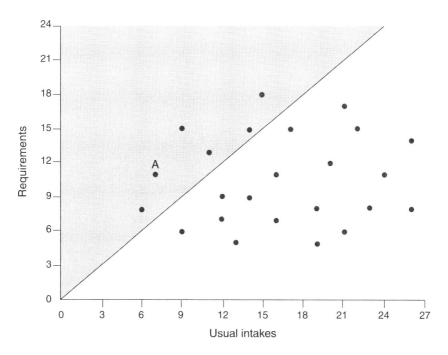

FIGURE 4-1 Plot of usual intakes and requirements of 24 hypothetical individuals in a group. The 45° line represents the points where nutrient intake equals nutrient requirement. Thus, the points to the right of the line are those individuals whose intakes are greater than their requirements. The points to the left of the line (the shaded area) are those individuals whose intakes are less than their requirements.

As before, the 45° line in Figure 4-2 denotes those individuals whose usual intake equals their own requirement. Determining the proportion of individuals in the population with inadequate intakes is simply done by counting how many points fall above the line (the shaded area).

*Note from this example: Even though the average usual intake is 25 percent higher than the average requirement (1,600 vs. 1,200 units), some people in the population still have intakes below their requirements. Simply comparing the average intake to the average requirement does **not** answer the question about how many in a group have inadequate intakes.*

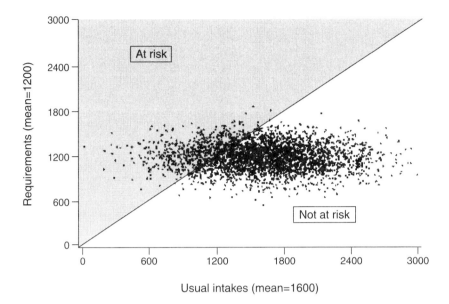

FIGURE 4-2 Plot of usual intakes and requirements of 3,000 hypothetical individuals in a population. By counting the points that fall to the left of the 45° line where intakes equal requirements (the shaded area), the proportion of the population with inadequate intakes can be determined.

Unfortunately, collecting data on the joint distribution of usual intake and requirements, such as those presented in Figures 4-1 and 4-2, is impractical because rarely is an individual's requirement known (if it were, it could be used to answer the question). Therefore, rather than observing the prevalence of inadequate intakes in the group, the prevalence can only be approximated by using other methods. The next two sections describe statistical approaches to estimating the prevalence of inadequate intakes—the probability approach (NRC, 1986) and a shortcut to the probability approach called the EAR cut-point method (Beaton, 1994; Carriquiry, 1999).

THE PROBABILITY APPROACH

The data typically available for nutrient assessment include estimated univariate distributions of usual intakes for a group of individuals and information from estimated univariate distributions of nutrient requirements of other groups that are similar to the group of interest. These univariate distributions can be combined and the prevalence of inadequate nutrient intakes can be estimated statistically by using the probability approach (NRC, 1986).

The probability approach relates individual intakes to the *distribution of requirements*. The probability approach applies a continuous risk-probability function to each individual's estimated intake and then averages the individual probabilities across the population or group. The first step in applying the probability approach is to construct a risk curve using the information on the requirement distribution of the group (median and variance). The risk curve specifies the probability that any given intake is inadequate for the individual consuming that intake. Figure 4-3 shows an example of a risk curve. An intake at the level of the average requirement has a probability of inadequacy of approximately 50 percent for all nutrients whose requirements follow a normal distribution.

The risk curve in Figure 4-3 is from a hypothetical nutrient requirement distribution. For simplicity, the requirements are normally distributed and the mean requirement is 100 units. Intake less than 50 units is associated with 100 percent risk of inadequacy whereas

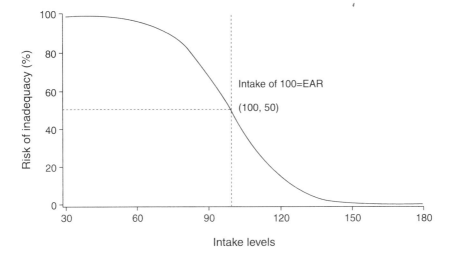

FIGURE 4-3 Risk curve from a normal requirement distribution having a mean of 100 units. Intakes less than 50 units are associated with 100 percent risk of inadequacy while intakes above 150 units have 0 percent risk of inadequacy. Intake equal to the mean requirement of 100 units has a 50 percent risk of inadequacy (the definition of the Estimated Average Requirement [EAR]).

intake greater than 150 is associated with 0 percent risk. As usual intake increases from 50 to 150 units, the risk of inadequacy associated with a specific intake declines.

The next step in the probability approach is to compare the risk curve to the distribution of usual intakes for the population to determine what proportion of the population has an inadequate intake. Figures 4-4 through 4-6 illustrate the relationship between the risk curve and the distribution of usual intakes in situations representing populations with high, medium, and low probabilities of inadequate intakes.

The example in Figure 4-4 shows what would happen when the usual intake distribution has a mean of about 50, and consists almost entirely of values less than 90. Because an intake of 90 units is associated with a risk of inadequacy of about 75 percent, almost all individuals in the population have intakes that reflect high risk of inadequacy. For a population with this distribution of intakes, the probability of inadequacy is—from visual inspection of the figure—very high. The average risk of inadequacy in this population is well above 75 percent as indicated in Figure 4-4 because the vast majority of intakes are below 90.

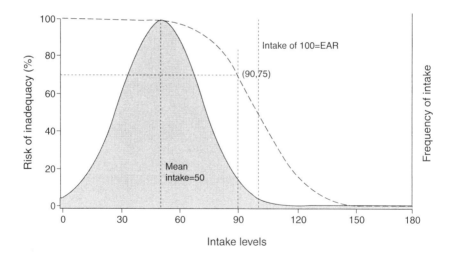

FIGURE 4-4 Risk curve combined with a usual intake distribution where the mean intake is less than the Estimated Average Requirement (EAR). The mean of the usual intake distribution is 50 units and the majority of the intake values are less than 90 units. At 90 units, the risk of inadequacy is about 75 percent. Therefore, in this population, the probability of inadequacy is high.

A second scenario shown in Figure 4-5 illustrates a different usual intake distribution with a mean of about 150 units and most of the values above 100. Most intakes fall to the right of the risk curve which translates to a lower population risk. Only individuals with intakes below 130 units (shaded area) have a risk of inadequacy above 5 percent.

More commonly though, a greater degree of overlap exists between the risk curve and the usual intake distribution. A more realistic example is provided in Figure 4-6. In this example, the usual intake distribution is for a population with a mean intake of 115 units and a standard deviation of 20 units. As expected, when the mean intake is 115 units and mean requirement is 100 units, some individuals are at risk of inadequacy (shaded area) and some are not. For example, about half of the population has a usual intake that exceeds 115 units, which is associated with a risk of 25 percent or less. An intake of 110 has about a 35 percent probability of inadequacy, an intake of 100 units (the median requirement) has about a 50 percent probability of inadequacy, and an intake of 80 units has about an 85 percent probability of inadequacy.

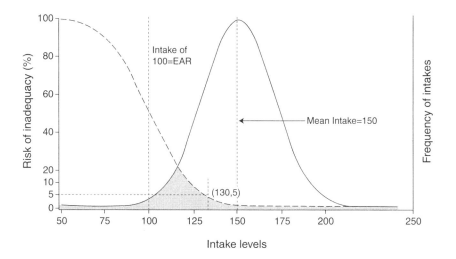

FIGURE 4-5 Risk curve combined with a usual intake distribution where the mean intake is much higher than the Estimated Average Requirement (EAR). Nearly the entire intake distribution falls to the right of the risk curve. Only those individuals in the population with intakes below 130 units have a risk of inadequate intake (shaded area).

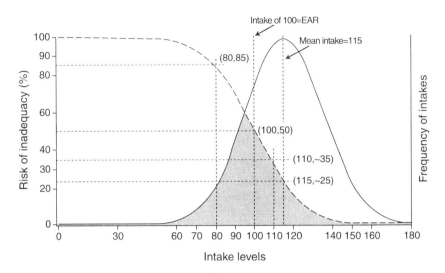

FIGURE 4-6 Risk curve combined with a usual intake distribution where mean intake (115 units) is slightly higher than the Estimated Average Requirement (EAR) (100 units). The risk curve and usual intake distribution have significant overlap. The proportion of individuals at risk of inadequacy (shaded area) at the mean intake is about 25 percent. The risk of inadequacy increases as intake becomes closer to the EAR.

Determining the prevalence of inadequate intakes for the population will depend on how many people have each particular value of intake and what the distribution of intakes looks like. Appendix C demonstrates how to carry out the necessary calculations to obtain a prevalence estimate for the group. Statistical programs (such as SAS or similar software) can be used to carry out these procedures.

Two key assumptions underlie the probability approach: (1) intakes and requirements are independent, and (2) the distribution of requirements is known. Frequently, it is assumed that the distribution of requirements is normal; however for some nutrients, such as iron for menstruating women, this assumption is not warranted (some women have very large menstrual losses of iron, which leads to a distribution that is positively skewed—i.e., more women have higher requirements than indicated by a normal distribution). For other nutrients the numbers of people for whom requirements have been experimentally determined is so small that it is just not possible to determine whether the assumption of normality is warranted (IOM, 1997, 1998b, 2000; NRC, 1986, 1989).

THE EAR CUT-POINT METHOD

The Estimated Average Requirement (EAR) cut-point method, proposed by Beaton (1994), is a shortcut derived from the probability approach described above. In contrast to the probability approach, the EAR cut-point method simply requires the distribution of requirements to be symmetrical. It is not necessary to know the actual variance of the requirement distribution, only its size relative to the intake variance. Like the probability approach, the EAR cut-point method requires knowledge of the median requirement (the EAR) for the nutrient and the distribution of usual intakes in the population.

Table 4-1 summarizes whether nutrients for which Dietary Reference Intakes (DRIs) have been established as of this writing (IOM, 1997, 1998b, 2000) meet the assumptions necessary to apply the EAR cut-point method for assessing the prevalence of inadequacy for groups.

The cut-point method is very simple. The population prevalence of inadequate intakes is computed as the proportion of the group

Box 4-1   The EAR cut-point method—what it is, and why it works

This method is very straightforward, and surprisingly, can sometimes be as accurate as the probability approach. With this method, the population prevalence of inadequate intakes is simply the proportion of the population with intakes below the median requirement (EAR). Modest departures from any of the assumptions listed below are likely to have only a small effect on the performance of the EAR cut-point method. However, the method does not work with nutrients such as energy where it is known that intakes and requirements are highly correlated, or with iron requirements in menstruating women where the requirement distribution is known to be highly skewed rather than symmetrical.

This method works well when:

- intakes are accurately measured
- actual prevalence in the group is neither very low nor very high
- estimated usual intakes of individuals are independent of each individual's requirement
- the distribution of requirements is approximately symmetrical
- variability in intakes among individuals in the group is greater than the variability in requirements of the individuals.

TABLE 4-1 Summary of Nutrients to Date with Dietary Reference Intakes (DRIs), and Whether They Meet the Assumptions Necessary to Apply the Estimated Average Requirement (EAR) Cut-Point Method for Assessing the Prevalence of Inadequacy for Groups

Established DRIs[a]

Nutrient	EAR	RDA	AI	UL
Magnesium	+	+		+
Phosphorus	+	+		+
Selenium	+	+		+
Thiamin	+	+		
Riboflavin	+	+		
Niacin	+	+		+
Vitamin B_6	+	+		+
Folate	+	+		+
Vitamin B_{12}	+	+		
Vitamin C	+	+		+
Vitamin E	+	+		+
Calcium			+	+
Fluoride			+	+
Biotin			+	
Choline			+	+
Vitamin D			+	+
Pantothenic Acid			+	

[a] RDA = Recommended Dietary Allowance; AI = Adequate Intake—the AI cannot be used with the EAR cut-point method; UL = Tolerable Upper Intake Level.
[b] Although there is little information on the variance of requirements, DRIs published to date have assumed a coefficient of variation (*CV*) of 10 or 15 percent. Variance of intake as calculated from the Continuing Survey of Food Intakes by Individuals 1994–

with intakes below the median requirement (EAR). In the example used when discussing the probability approach, population prevalence according to the EAR cut-point method would be the proportion of individuals with usual intakes below 100 units, the EAR.

Figure 4-7 illustrates the EAR cut-point method. The shaded area corresponds to the proportion of individuals in the group whose intakes are less than the EAR and the unshaded area corresponds to the proportion with usual intakes greater than the EAR. A discussion of why this approach works follows.

Meets the Assumptions of the Cut-Point Method			
Variance of Intake is Greater than Variance of Requirement[b]	Requirement Distribution Symmetrical[c]	Intake and Requirement Independent or Have Low Correlation	CV of the Requirement[d] (%)
Yes	Assumed	Yes	10
Yes	Assumed	Yes	10
Yes	Assumed	Yes	10
Yes	Assumed	Yes	10
Yes	Assumed	Yes	10
Yes	Assumed	Yes	15
Yes	Assumed	Yes	10
Yes	Assumed	Yes	10
Yes	Assumed	Yes	10
Yes	Assumed	Yes	10
Yes	Assumed	Yes	10

1996 indicates that for all nutrients, intake variance is well above the assumed requirement variance.

[c] Data to determine the shape of requirement distributions are lacking for most nutrients; therefore, symmetry is assumed unless there are data adequate to indicate otherwise.

[d] CV of the requirement is needed for the probability approach.

Figure 4-8 shows the same hypothetical (simulated) joint distribution of intakes and requirements for the group of individuals presented in Figure 4-2. The figure includes joint intake and requirement data from 3,000 people, with a mean intake of 1,600 units and a mean requirement of 1,200 units. As before, intakes and requirements are independent (i.e., individuals with higher intakes are not more likely to have higher requirements).

As discussed earlier, the proportion of the population with inadequate intakes could be obtained simply by counting the people who

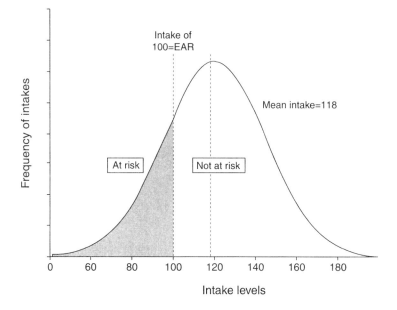

FIGURE 4-7 The Estimated Average Requirement (EAR) cut-point method. The shaded area represents the proportion of individuals in the group whose intakes are below the EAR, while the unshaded area represents the proportion with usual intakes above the EAR.

were above the 45° line. Most of the people who do not meet their requirements have intakes below 1,200 units—the median requirement, denoted in Figure 4-8 by the vertical line labeled intake = EAR. However, some individuals who have intakes greater than the EAR are still below their own individual requirements. The points for these individuals fall within the triangle-shaped area (referred to here as a triangle) A in Figure 4-8, bounded by the intake = EAR line and the 45° line to the right of the intake = EAR line. Conversely, some of the people who have intakes less than the EAR do not have inadequate intakes—even though their intakes are below the median requirement of the group, they are still exceeding their individual requirements. The points for these people fall within triangle B in Figure 4-8, bounded by the intake = EAR line and the 45° line to the left of the intake = EAR line.

Unfortunately, it is very difficult to identify individuals represented by points in triangle A (intake greater than the EAR but less than the individual requirement), because information would be needed

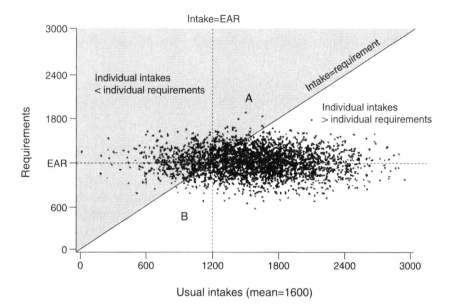

FIGURE 4-8 Joint distribution of intakes and requirements from a hypothetical population of 3,000 individuals. Intakes are independent of requirements. The mean intake is 1,600 units and the median requirement (Estimated Average Requirement [EAR]) is 1,200 units. The triangle labeled A is bounded by the intake = EAR line and the 45° line where intake = requirement. Points above the 45° line (shaded area), represent those individuals whose intakes are above the EAR, but below their own individual requirement. Individuals in triangle B have intakes below the EAR, yet above their own requirement. The number of people in triangle A is approximately equal to the number in triangle B.

on both their usual intake and their requirement and such information is rarely available. A similar number of individuals are represented by points in triangle A and in triangle B, and therefore the number above the 45° line (where intake = requirement) can be approximated by counting the number to the left of the intake = EAR line. Essentially, the EAR cut-point method substitutes the individuals in B for the individuals in A. It is easier to count the number of individuals to the left of the intake = EAR line than those above the 45° line because this only requires information on each individual's intake. Therefore, to use this method, the only information required is each individual's usual intake of the nutrient and the EAR of the group; individual requirements are not needed.

Because the number of people in triangle A is approximately equal to the number in triangle B, these two groups cancel each other out, and the proportion of the population above the 45° line (inadequate intakes, shaded area of graph) is approximately equal to the proportion of the population to the left of the intake = EAR line. In other words, the proportion of the population with intakes below their requirements (from the joint distribution approach) is about the same as the proportion of the population with intakes less than the EAR, even though some of the individuals in these two groups are not the same.

Box 4-2   *The EAR cut-point method—when it works*

The EAR cut-point method works best (produces an almost unbiased estimate of prevalence of nutrient inadequacy) when:

1. intakes and requirements are independent
2. the requirement distribution is symmetrical around the EAR
3. the variance in intakes is larger than the variance of requirements
4. true prevalence of inadequacy in the population is no smaller than 8 to 10 percent or no larger than 90 to 92 percent.

If the true prevalence in the group is about 50 percent—so that the mean intake is approximately equal to the EAR—then the EAR cut-point method results in almost unbiased estimates of prevalence of inadequacy even if conditions 1 and 3 are not met (see Appendix D).[1]

The EAR cut-point method—when it does not work

What happens when the assumptions required for the cut-point method are not met? In the following section, examples are provided of situations in which the assumptions do not hold. The cut-point method can either underestimate or overestimate the population prevalence of inadequacy under such circumstances.

---

[1] Estimates of prevalence of inadequacy obtained using the EAR cut-point method are, by construction, slightly biased except when the mean intake and the EAR are similar. The relative bias in the prevalence estimate increases as the difference between the mean intake in the group and the EAR of the nutrient increases. When true prevalence of inadequacy in the group is moderate (perhaps no less than 10 percent), the bias in the estimate arising from the EAR cut-point method is negligible as long as the conditions listed above are met. When true prevalence in the group is very small (perhaps between 1 and 3 percent), the relative bias can be very large—that is, the EAR cut-point method may result in an estimate of prevalence of 3 percent when the true prevalence is 1 or 2 percent.

The results of some preliminary simulation studies conducted to assess the performance of the EAR cut-point method in different situations are presented in Appendix D.

What Happens if Intakes and Requirements Are Not Independent?

Intakes for certain nutrients—energy for example—increase with increased needs. This leads to a situation in which individuals with higher requirements usually have higher intakes. In other words, requirements and intakes are correlated rather than independent.

The implications of this correlation for estimating the proportion of a population with inadequate intakes can be observed in Figure 4-9, which shows the scatter plot of usual intakes and requirements sloping upward, reflecting a positive correlation between intake and requirement. Note the number of data points in triangle A, which

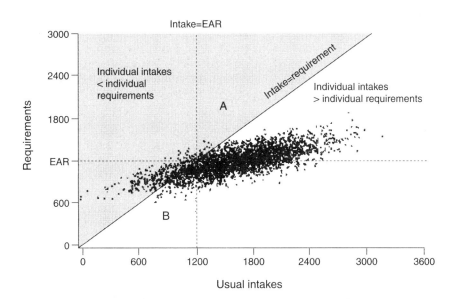

FIGURE 4-9 Intakes and requirements are positively correlated. In this scenario, the number of individuals in triangle A is less than the number in triangle B. Using the Estimated Average Requirement (EAR) cut-point method would *overestimate* the number of people with inadequate intakes.

represent individuals with intakes greater than the EAR, who still do not meet their requirements (they are to the right of the intake = EAR line in the shaded area above the 45° line where intake equals requirement). Next, note the number of data points in triangle B which represent individuals with intakes below the EAR but whose intakes are adequate. The EAR cut-point method works when intakes and requirements are independent (see Figure 4-8) and the number of points in triangles A and B are virtually identical. In Figure 4-9 there are more points in triangle B than in triangle A. Accordingly, when usual intake and requirement are correlated, using the EAR cut-point method (i.e., determining the number of individuals to the left of the intake = EAR line) would *overestimate* the number of people with inadequate intakes (those in the shaded area above the 45° line where intake = requirement).

This example is illustrative, but does not indicate what the expected bias resulting from using the cut-point method might be. The bias of the cut-point method will be severe for energy because the correlation between usual energy intakes and requirements (expenditure) is high. How severe a bias is expected if the association between intakes and requirements is not as extreme? This question is difficult to answer because usual intakes and requirements cannot be observed for a sufficiently large sample of individuals. However, limited empirical evidence suggests that the expected bias is likely to be low as long as the correlation between intakes and requirements is moderate—no larger than 0.25 or 0.30 (Carriquiry, 1999). Furthermore, when the mean intake of a group and the EAR are approximately the same, the effect of the correlation on the bias of the cut-point method is likely to be very low even at correlations greater than 0.30. An exception to this rule is the extreme case in which the correlation between intakes and requirements of the nutrient is equal to 1. In this unlikely event, the prevalence estimates obtained from the EAR cut-point method will be severely biased, even if mean intake and the EAR are identical. This purely hypothetical case is used in an illustrative example in the next section.

Do the probability approach and the EAR cut-point method work for food energy?

No, because empirical evidence indicates a strong correlation between energy intake and energy requirements. This correlation most likely reflects either the regulation of energy intake to meet needs or the adjustment of energy expenditures to be consistent with intakes (FAO/WHO/UNU, 1985). Because of this strong correlation, neither the EAR cut-point method nor the probability approach can be used to assess the probability of inadequacy of food energy intake.

The problem with using the EAR cut-point method for food energy can best be illustrated by considering an admittedly extreme example of both a perfect correlation between individual intakes and requirements and mean intake equal to the average requirement. Because each individual in the group has a usual intake equal to his or her requirement, the prevalence of inadequacy is zero. However, because one-half of the group has usual intakes less than the average requirement and one-half has usual intakes exceeding the average requirement, the cut-point method would estimate that 50 percent of the group is at risk of inadequate intakes when, in fact, the prevalence of inadequacy is zero.

Therefore, to assess energy adequacy, information other than intakes could be used, such as body weight for height, body mass index, or other anthropometric measures.

Situations in which nutrient intakes and requirements may be related to a third variable (e.g., energy and thiamin, body weight and protein) have not been well studied.

What Happens if the Requirement Distribution Is Not Symmetrical?

A good example of an asymmetrical requirement distribution is iron requirements in menstruating women. The iron requirement includes the need to replace urine, fecal, and dermal iron losses, and this aspect of the requirement does appear to be symmetrically distributed in the population (FAO/WHO, 1988). For menstruating women, iron lost in menstrual flow varies considerably—the mean loss averaged over 1 month has been estimated at 0.5 mg/day but about 5 percent of women have losses averaging more than 1.4 mg/day (FAO/WHO, 1988; Hallberg et al., 1966). This means that the distribution of iron requirements in women is skewed—there are more women with needs 25 percent or more above the mean, for example, than with needs 25 percent or more below the mean. In this case, the mean requirement is different from the median requirement (or EAR) in the group.

Figure 4-10 illustrates this situation, which is modeled after the information about iron requirements in women given in the FAO/WHO report of 1988. The median requirement (EAR) is 10 mg but the distribution of requirements is not symmetrical around the

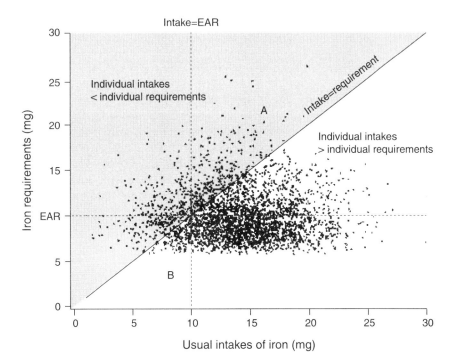

FIGURE 4-10 The distribution of requirements is not symmetrical. In this example, the number of individuals in triangle A is greater than the number in triangle B. The Estimated Average Requirement (EAR) cut-point method would result in an underestimate of the true prevalence of inadequacy. The shaded area represents individuals with usual intakes less than their requirements. The unshaded area represents individuals with usual intakes greater than their requirements.

10 mg median horizontal line; virtually no one has a requirement below about 6 mg but many have requirements above 14 mg (a similar distance from the median requirement of 10 mg). Put another way, there is a greater spread of requirements above than below the median.

In this example, more individuals are represented by points that fall in the shaded area above the 45° line where intake = requirement (and hence have inadequate intakes) than fall to the left of the intake = EAR line, where they would be estimated as being at risk by the EAR cut-point method. To continue using the triangle approach, the number of points in triangle A (greater than the EAR but still inadequate [shaded area]) is considerably greater than the number in triangle B (less than the EAR but adequate). Thus, when the distribution of requirement is skewed, the EAR cut-point method results in a biased estimate (in this case, an *underestimate*) of the true prevalence of inadequacy.

For which nutrients are the requirement distribution not symmetrical?

One nutrient for which it is known that requirements are not symmetrical about the EAR is iron in menstruating women. Because requirement data are so scarce, it is often difficult to investigate the shape of the distribution of requirements for every nutrient in every life stage and gender group. Indeed, there is virtually no information on the actual characteristics of any requirement distributions except perhaps protein in adult men and iron in adult women (FAO/WHO, 1988; FAO/WHO/UNU, 1985).

In the absence of additional information about the shape of the requirement distribution of a nutrient, it is implicitly assumed in this report (and the DRI nutrient reports) that the unknown distribution is symmetrical around the median requirement (the EAR).

When it is known that the distribution of requirements is skewed, the full probability approach can be used by computing a risk curve that reflects the skewed requirements. The FAO/WHO (1988) adopted a log normal distribution to model iron requirements in women and applied the probability approach under the log normal assumption.

The effect of skewness on the bias of the EAR cut-point method is likely to be significant. Even moderate amounts of skewness in the distribution of requirements may result in noticeable biases in prevalence estimates with the cut-point method. Therefore, when the distribution of requirements is known to be asymmetrical, as for iron in menstruating women, the probability approach, not the EAR cut-point method, is recommended for assessing the prevalence of nutrient inadequacy.

What Happens if the Variance of Requirement Is Greater Than the Variance of Intake?

At least in North America, the situation where variation in individual requirements is greater than variation in individual usual intakes is most likely to arise for institutionalized subpopulations— for example, prison inmates or residents of a long-term care facility—who are all fed similar diets. Figure 4-11 illustrates this scenario:

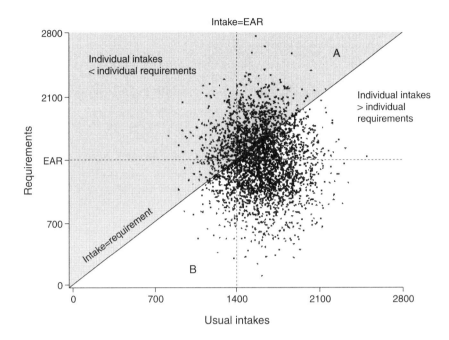

FIGURE 4-11 The variance of requirements is greater than the variance of intakes. In this case, the number of individuals in triangle A is greater than the number in B. The Estimated Average Requirement (EAR) cut-point method would underestimate the true prevalence of inadequacy. Points in the shaded area represent individuals with usual intakes below their requirements while points in the unshaded area represent individuals with usual intake above their requirements.

the median requirement (EAR) has been set at 1,400 units and the mean of the usual intake distribution has been set at 1,600 units. Note that although the mean intake exceeds the median requirement, there is much more spread in requirements than there is in intake.

The proportion of the population with inadequate intake (i.e., points in the shaded area above the 45° line where intake = requirement) is not the same as the proportion whose intake falls to the left of the intake = EAR line (estimated as being at risk using the cut-point method). The number of points in triangles A and B is different, with more points in triangle A than in triangle B. This means that the cut-point method, in this example, would *underestimate* the proportion of the population with inadequate intakes.

The bias resulting from the use of the cut-point method here is rather noticeable; thus, caution needs to be exercised when using the EAR cut-point method in situations in which requirements for a nutrient may be more variable than intakes of the nutrient.

The extent and direction of the bias that occurs when requirements are more variable than intakes will differ depending on whether the mean intake is above (as in Figure 4-11), equal to, or below the mean requirement. Carriquiry (1999) assessed the expected bias in several of these scenarios using a limited simulation study in which the relative sizes and standard deviations of the mean intake and the mean requirement were varied. The results suggest that in situations where the variance of requirement exceeds the variance of usual intake, the following cases arise:

1. When mean intake equals median requirement, use of the EAR cut-point method accurately estimates the proportion of the population with inadequate intakes.

2. When mean intake exceeds median requirement, use of the EAR cut-point method *underestimates* the proportion with inadequate nutrient intake.

3. When mean intake is less than median requirement, use of the EAR cut-point method *overestimates* the proportion with inadequate nutrient intake.

4. In the last two cases, the bias in the prevalence estimate can be significant even when the standard deviation of requirements is only slightly larger than the variation of usual intakes. The over- or underestimation of true prevalence is more pronounced when the true prevalence in the group is either very low or very high.

ADJUSTING INTAKE DISTRIBUTIONS

Regardless of the method chosen to assess prevalence of inadequate nutrient intakes in a group of individuals, information is required about the distribution of intakes of the nutrient in the group. Because the chronic effect of diet on an individual's well being is often of interest, the estimation of the distribution of long-term average intakes—that is, usual intakes—for the group is a concern. The usual intake distribution of a dietary component should have a spread (or variance) that reflects the individual-to-individual variation of intakes of that nutrient within the group.

Usual intake distributions can be estimated by adjusting the distribution of the mean of a few days of intake of each individual in the group. This general method was proposed by the National Research

Council (NRC, 1986) and was further developed by Nusser et al. (1996). As described below, to apply these methods of adjusting intake distributions it is necessary to have at least two independent 24-hour recalls or diet records for at least some individuals in the group (or at least three days when data are collected over consecutive days). Independent observations are obtained by collecting intake data over nonconsecutive days.

Reasons for Adjusting Intake Distributions

Several characteristics of dietary intake data make estimating the distribution of usual intakes for a group a challenging problem. This section focuses on the need for adjustment of distributions, illustrates the use of two of the most widely used approaches, and discusses the consequences of poorly estimating usual intake distributions.

Dietary intake data have characteristics that need to be taken into account when estimating the usual intake distribution of a nutrient for a group of individuals. If intake distributions are not properly adjusted, the prevalence of nutrient inadequacy will either be overestimated or underestimated, regardless of whether the probability approach or the cut-point method is chosen.

Should the distribution of observed intakes be used as an estimate of the usual intake distribution?

No. Although the mean *of the distribution of observed intakes in the group is an unbiased estimate of the mean usual intake in that group (assuming that intakes have been accurately measured), the* variance *of the distribution of observed intakes is almost always too large (NRC, 1986; Nusser et al., 1996). This is because it includes both the within-person (day-to-day) variation and the individual-to-individual variation, thus leading to estimates of prevalence of inadequacy or excess that are likely to be higher than the true prevalence. In order to get accurate prevalence estimates, the distribution of observed intakes must be adjusted to more closely reflect only the individual-to-individual variability in intakes.*

Large Within-Person Variation in Intakes

Individuals usually vary the types and amounts of the foods they consume from day to day. This translates into a large variability in the within-person intake of nutrients. For some nutrients, more within-person (or day-to-day) variation than between-person variation may occur. Vitamin A is a good example of this. Intake can be 5,000 retinol equivalents (RE) on a day when the individual snacked on carrots, and close to 0 RE on another day when few fruits, vegetables, and dairy products were consumed. Thus, for some nutrients, the day-to-day variability in intakes for an individual may be larger than the between-person variability in the group. For vitamin A, the within-person variability in intakes may be as much as six times larger than the between-person variability in intakes in typical North American dietary data (Basiotis et al., 1987). For other dietary components such as energy, the day-to-day variability in intakes is about as large as the between-person variability in intakes in the group (Basiotis et al., 1987; Beaton et al., 1983; Guenther et al., 1997; Liu et al., 1978; Looker et al., 1990; NRC, 1986; Nusser et al., 1996; Sempos et al., 1985). This means that if the aim is to estimate the usual intake distribution of a nutrient in a group and have its spread reflect only the between-person variation in intakes, then statistical methods that help reduce this nuisance variance must be used.

Heterogeneous Within-Person Variation in Intakes

Not only do individual intakes differ from day to day, as discussed above, but also how much they differ varies from one person to another. In addition, this variability is not completely random. Individuals with higher average intakes also tend to have more variable intakes than do individuals with lower average intakes (Nusser et al., 1996).

Skewed Intake Distributions

For most nutrients, the distribution of observed mean intakes (and presumably, the usual intake distribution as well) is skewed to the high end rather than being symmetrical. This is particularly true when intakes from supplements are included in the diet. Consider calcium as an example. Mean intake in a group might be 600 mg/day. Very few people would have intakes 500 mg or more below the mean (and it would be impossible to have an intake more than 600 mg below the mean), but there could easily be people in the group consuming intakes 500, 1,000, or even 1,500 mg above the mean. Therefore, the intake of this nutrient has a skewed, asymmetrical distribution. Because most nutrients have skewed, asymmetrical intake distributions, statistical procedures that assume that nutrient intake data are normally distributed cannot be applied to these data.

Day-to-Day Correlation in Intake Data Collected over Consecutive Days

When intake data are collected over consecutive days, observations for an individual cannot be assumed to be independent because what is consumed on one day often affects what is consumed on the next. This effect can work several ways—the same meal may be repeated the next day (as with leftovers) or the same food may be avoided two days in a row (as with liver). In either case, the assumption of independence for within-person observations does not hold unless dietary intake data are collected several days apart. The length of time needed between observations so that independence can be assumed depends on the dietary component. For energy, for example, it suffices to space daily observations one or two days apart, but for vitamin A, which is not present in all foods, a three- to four-day gap between 24-hour recalls for the same individual might be necessary to guarantee independence among observations.

Other Survey-Related or Nuisance Effects

Dietary intake data are often collected in nationwide food consumption surveys that have a complex design and response rates under 100 percent. In these cases, each respondent carries a sampling weight that corrects that individual's importance in the sample. These weights must be carried throughout the procedure for estimating usual intake distributions if this estimated distribution is to be used to make inferences about the wider population from which the group was drawn.

Overview of Methods to Adjust Mean Intake Distributions

Because of the above attributes of dietary intake data, obtaining reliable estimates of usual intake distributions is not straightforward. The NRC, in its 1986 report, set forth the concept of a usual intake distribution, and proposed a statistical approach to adjust observed mean intake distributions to partially remove the day-to-day variability in intakes. The resulting estimated usual intake distribution has a spread that approximately reflects the between-individual variability in intakes (NRC, 1986). Aickin and Ritenbaugh (1991) proposed an algorithm—called the unmixing algorithm—for adjusting vitamin A intake distributions. Nusser and colleagues (1996), Stefanski and Bay (1996), Eckert and coworkers (1997), and more recently Chen (1999) started from the method proposed by the NRC (1986) and suggested methods for estimating usual intake distributions that address different sets of characteristics of dietary intake data. Brief descriptions of two approaches, the NRC (1986) method and the method developed at Iowa State University (ISU method, Nusser et al., 1996) are provided because they are most used today (Beaton, 1994; Carriquiry et al., 1997).

Suppose that daily intake data for a group of individuals are available. These data may have been collected via 24-hour recall methods or perhaps from multiple-day diet records. For each of the individuals, multiple days of dietary intake data were recorded. Even though it is assumed here that each individual in the group has the same number of independent daily intake observations, neither of the methods described below require that each individual in the group have the same number of observations. It is possible to adjust intake distributions as long as *some* individuals in the group have two or more daily intake observations, even if for many of the individuals only one observation is available.

For multiple daily intake observations for each individual in the sample, it is possible to obtain, for each individual, the mean intake over the multiple days of recording. As is discussed in Chapter 3, observed mean intakes can be used as estimates of individual usual intake, albeit imprecise ones. *Estimating the usual intake distribution in the group as the distribution of the observed mean intakes, however intuitively appealing, is incorrect.* The individual daily intakes must be used, rather than the mean intake, in order to adjust the usual intake distribution.

The National Research Council Method to Adjust Intake Distributions

In recognizing that daily intakes for an individual vary from day to day, and that daily intake data are not normally distributed, the NRC (1986) proposed that day-to-day variability in intakes be partially removed by fitting a measurement error model to daily intake data which had been power transformed. Power transformation refers to a family of mathematical conversions that includes, for example, the square root, the cube root, and log transformations (Fuller, 1987). The power transformation reduces the skewness typically observed in the distribution of daily intakes. The measurement error model establishes that, in the transformed scale, the nutrient intake observed for an individual on a day is a deviation from that individual's usual intake of the nutrient. That is,

(transformed) observed intake = usual intake + deviation from usual intake.

The simple model above is called a measurement error model (Fuller, 1987), because it states that observed intakes measure usual intakes with error. Measurement error, in a statistical sense, denotes a (random) deviation from a variable of interest—in this case the usual intake. The error is modeled as a random variable with zero mean and with a variance that reflects the day-to-day variability in intakes.

The adjustment described by the NRC method is relatively straightforward to implement, once the magnitude of the day-to-day variation in intake has been determined for the group. After any necessary transformations to ensure normality, the difference between each person's intake and the mean intake of the group is multiplied by the ratio of day-to-day variation to the total variation, and then added back to the mean intake for the group. These adjusted intakes can then be transformed back to the original scale, as appropriate, and used for further analyses.

In the NRC method the variance of the measurement error was assumed to be constant across individuals. This means that the NRC method establishes that the day-to-day variability in intakes is constant across individuals. A more general version of this basic method developed at ISU by Nusser and colleagues (1996) does not require the measurement error variance to be constant across individuals.

The Iowa State University Method to Adjust Intake Distributions

In general, the statistical method developed at ISU (Nusser et al., 1996) elaborates on the NRC method and produces estimates of usual intake distributions with good statistical properties. Details about the procedure can be found elsewhere (Guenther et al., 1997; Nusser et al., 1996). The following example illustrates how its use can affect the conclusions drawn when a dietary survey is used to assess intakes for a group.

How large a sample size, and what proportion of replicate observations are needed for the ISU method of estimating usual nutrient intake distributions? An exact answer to this question is difficult to provide. Regarding actual sample size, the performance of the ISU method improves as sample size increases; small sample sizes of fewer than about 50 or 60 individuals result in unreliable estimates of usual intake distributions (Nusser et al., 1996). Because only the replicate observations in the sample contain information about the day-to-day variability in intakes, it is important to have a moderately large number of individuals in the replicate sample, perhaps not fewer than 30 or 40, and these individuals should be representative of the full group. Each person in this sample must have at least two independent daily intake measurements or three daily intake measurements if data are collected on consecutive days.

Carriquiry and colleagues (1997) successfully applied the ISU method to adjust intake distributions and distributions of blood biochemical measurements using data collected in the Third National Health and Nutrition Examination Survey (NHANES III), even though sample sizes for some life stage and gender groups were moderately small (fewer than 70 to 80 individuals) and the proportion of replicate observations was low (approximately 6 percent). In general however, having a minimum *number* of replicate records in the sample is more important than having a minimum *proportion* of replicate observations.

The following example is based on estimated usual intake distributions for two dietary components—phosphorus and vitamin B_6— for women aged 19 through 50 years who were neither pregnant nor lactating at the time the data were collected. Only intakes from food were considered (i.e., intake from supplements is not included in these examples). The dietary intake data were collected in NHANES III, so only a small proportion of individuals in the sample had a replicate observation collected several weeks after the first. Estimated Average Requirements (EARs) have been established for the two nutrients in this example (IOM, 1997, 1998b). Using the EAR cut-point method, the proportion of women at risk of nutrient inadequacy can be estimated by computing the percentage of individuals in the group with usual intakes below the corresponding EAR.

For purposes of illustration, the usual intake distributions of phosphorus and vitamin B_6 were estimated by two different approaches: (1) using only the first day of intake data for each individual in the sample; and (2) using replicate intake data (whenever available) and applying the ISU method to adjust the distribution. It is anticipated that the estimate of the usual intake distribution obtained using one day of intake data will have the incorrect variance; the variance of the estimated distribution will contain an unwanted day-to-day variability component. Therefore, estimates of the prevalence of nutrient inadequacy will be biased. The two estimates of the usual intake distribution are shown in Figure 4-12 for vitamin B$_6$ and Figure 4-13 for phosphorus.

The adjusted estimate of the usual intake distribution has a smaller variance than does the estimate obtained using one day of intake data. This is to be expected because one of the features of the method (and also of the method proposed by NRC) is that it partially removes the day-to-day variability in intakes. Thus, the estimated usual intake distribution obtained by applying the adjustment has a variance that reflects only the between-person variability in intakes, whereas the estimate obtained using one-day data has a variance that is inflated by day-to-day variability.

The shapes of the two distributions in Figure 4-12 are quite different. More importantly, the conclusions drawn about the proportion of individuals in the group whose intakes of vitamin B$_6$ are inadequate also differ, depending on which estimate of the usual intake

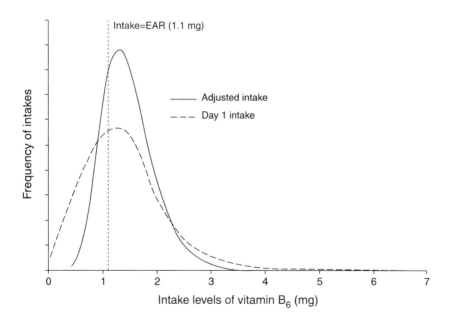

FIGURE 4-12 Estimates of a usual intake distribution of vitamin B$_6$ obtained from one day of intake data and adjusted using replicate intake data via the Iowa State University method. The *y*-axis shows the likelihood of each level of intake in the population.

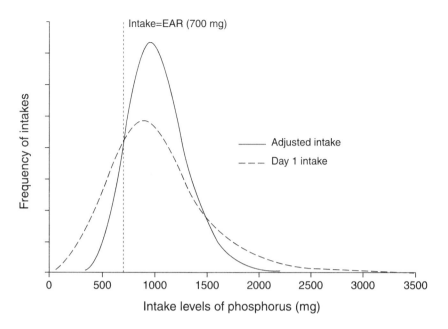

FIGURE 4-13 Estimates of a usual intake distribution of phosphorus obtained from one day of intake data and adjusted using replicate intake data via the Iowa State University method. The y-axis shows the likelihood of each level of intake in the population.

distribution is used. As was discussed previously, the prevalence of nutrient inadequacy in a group is estimated as the proportion of individuals in the group whose usual intakes are below the EAR established for the nutrient. The vertical line in Figure 4-12 represents the intake level that is equal to the EAR for vitamin B₆ for women ages 19 through 50 years; this value is 1.1 mg/day (IOM, 1998b).

If only one day of intake data is available for each individual in the sample and therefore adjusting the intake distribution to remove day-to-day variability in intakes is not possible, the estimate of prevalence of inadequacy in this group of women is 37 percent. If, instead, the prevalence estimate is based on the adjusted distribution, the conclusion is that 23 percent of women are not consuming an adequate amount of vitamin B₆. The 14 percent difference between the two estimates is due exclusively to the method used to estimate the usual intake distribution. Using a single day of intake data for each individual in the sample is indefensible from a statistical viewpoint if the objective is to estimate prevalence of inadequacy.

Results from the same analyses applied to phosphorus intakes are shown in Figure 4-13. For phosphorus, prevalence of inadequacy estimates computed from the one-day and the adjusted intake distributions are 25 and 11 percent, respectively.

In these two cases (where the means of the intake distributions are greater than the EAR), the bias in the prevalence estimate that results from not removing the day-to-day variability in intakes leads to an *overestimation* of the proportion of individuals in the group whose intakes are inadequate. This is not always so; if the mean of the usual intake distribution is less than the EAR, using the one-day distribution to estimate prevalence may result in *underestimation*.

INAPPROPRIATE APPROACHES FOR GROUP-LEVEL ASSESSMENT USING THE RDA

Should the Recommended Dietary Allowance (RDA) be used to assess the proportion of individuals in a group who are at risk of nutrient inadequacy?

No.
Estimating prevalence of nutrient inadequacy in a group by computing the proportion in the group with intakes below the RDA always leads to an overestimation of the true prevalence of inadequacy.

By definition, the RDA is the intake level that exceeds the requirements of a large proportion of individuals in the group. In fact, when requirements in the population are distributed as normal random variables, the RDA exceeds the requirement of more than 97 percent of all individuals in the group.

As indicated previously in this chapter, the proportion of individuals in a group with nutrient intakes below their requirements can be estimated by using the Estimated Average Requirement (EAR) cut-point method (calculating the proportion of individuals in the group with intakes below the EAR). Examples were presented in which the cut-point method was shown to perform well. That is, when populations were simulated for which both nutrient intakes and requirements were known, approximately the same prevalence estimates resulted either by counting the actual number of individuals with nutrient intakes below their requirements or the number of individuals with intakes less than the EAR.

It is evident, then, that comparing usual nutrient intakes with the RDA, which by construction is always larger than the EAR (i.e., RDA = EAR + 2 standard deviations of requirements), will lead to estimates of inadequacy that are too large.

Comparing Group Mean Intakes with a Percentage of a Reference Value

Some of the most common mistakes in evaluating dietary data arise from comparisons of mean intakes with RDAs. In particular, when studies find group mean intakes equal to or exceeding the RDA, the conclusion has often been that group diets are adequate and conform to recognized nutritional standards. Sometimes, group-mean intake is even compared with some percentage of the RDA. However, these comparisons are inappropriate and may result in very misleading conclusions.

For most nutrients (except food energy), group mean intake must exceed the RDA for there to be an acceptably low prevalence of inadequate intakes. To achieve a low prevalence of inadequate intakes (e.g., such that almost all individuals would meet their requirements), the group-mean intake would need to be equal to the EAR plus two standard deviations of intake (when intakes are normally distributed). Recall that the variability of intakes usually exceeds the variability in requirements and that the RDA is equal to the EAR plus two standard deviations of requirement. Thus the group mean intake needed for there to be a low prevalence of inadequate intake must exceed the RDA. The greater the variability in usual intakes relative to variability in requirements, the greater the mean intake must be relative to the RDA to ensure that only a small proportion of the group has inadequate intakes.

It follows from the above discussion that if the group mean intake equals the RDA, a substantial proportion of the group will have intakes less than their own requirements. Even if mean intake exceeds the RDA, there may be a substantial proportion of a group with intakes less than requirements.

An even stronger caution is needed when comparing group mean intakes with the EAR. If mean intake equals the average requirement (EAR), a very high proportion of the population will have inadequate usual intake. In fact, roughly half the population is expected to have intake less than requirement (except for energy).

In summary, except for food energy, group-mean intakes must exceed the RDA to have a relatively low prevalence of inadequate intakes. In general, however, group mean intakes should not be used to assess the prevalence of inadequate dietary intakes. It is far preferable to use the EAR cut-point method and the adjusted distribution of usual intakes to estimate the proportion of a group with inadequate intakes.

UNITS OF OBSERVATION OTHER THAN THE INDIVIDUAL

In the preceding discussion, the unit of observation implicitly assumed in the dietary assessment is the individual. What if the unit of observation is either the household or the population? Consumption data are frequently gathered for households rather than for individuals. Disappearance data (or food balance sheets) may be collected for a group or an entire population such as a country. However, published requirement estimates usually are related to individuals. For dietary assessment applications, however, estimates of nutrient requirements and nutrient intakes must be at the same level of aggregation: individual, household, or population. Appendix E suggests approaches for evaluating dietary adequacy when the unit of observation is not the individual.

SUMMARY

Assessing the proportion of a group or population that is at risk of nutrient inadequacy is an important public health and policy concern. The Dietary Reference Intake (DRI) that is relevant to this type of assessment is the Estimated Average Requirement (EAR). The probability approach, described by the National Research Council (NRC) in 1986, permits an estimation of the prevalence of inadequacy within a group by comparing intakes with the distribution of requirements. This method assumes that the correlation between intake and requirement is low and that the distribution of requirements is known. A shortcut to the probability approach—the EAR cut-point method—allows determination of the prevalence of inadequacy in a group by determining the number of individuals with intakes below the EAR. Like the probability approach, the cut-point method assumes that the correlation between intake and requirement is low and that the variability in intakes is greater than the variability of requirements. However, unlike the probability approach, the cut-point method does not require that the actual shape of the requirement distribution be known, but does require that the distribution be symmetrical. Examples demonstrated the biases that occur when the assumptions of the cut-point method are violated. Assessing the prevalence of inadequacy of iron intake in women requires use of the probability approach because of the highly skewed nature of the requirement distribution. Because of the very high correlation between intakes and requirements, energy is the one nutrient for which neither the probability approach nor the cut-point method can be used to assess adequacy. The prevalence of nutrient inadequacy for a group will usually be overestimated by either method if dietary intake data are not adjusted for day-to-day within-person variation. Thus, a minimum of two nonconsecutive or three consecutive days of intake data on at least a representative sample of the group is needed for dietary assessment of groups.

5

Using the Adequate Intake for Nutrient Assessment of Groups

This chapter briefly describes the inherent limitations of the Adequate Intake (AI) as a Dietary Reference Intake, and its limited application in assessing nutrient adequacy of groups.

DERIVATIONS OF THE AI

How is the Adequate Intake (AI) defined?

The AI is a recommended average daily nutrient intake level, based on experimentally derived intake levels or approximations of observed mean nutrient intake by a group (or groups) of apparently healthy people that are assumed to be adequate.

An AI is established when there is insufficient scientific evidence to determine an Estimated Average Requirement (EAR). In the judgment of the Standing Committee on the Scientific Evaluation of Dietary Reference Intakes, the AI is expected to meet or exceed the amount needed to maintain a defined nutritional state or criterion of adequacy in essentially all members of a specific apparently healthy population. Examples of defined nutritional states include normal growth, maintenance of normal circulating nutrient values, or other aspects of nutritional well-being or general health. The AI is developed as a guide for individuals about an appropriate level of intake for nutrients for which data are insufficient to establish a requirement.

When the AI is based on observed mean intakes of population groups, it is likely to always exceed the average requirement that would have been experimentally determined.

In the Dietary Reference Intake (DRI) nutrient reports (IOM, 1997, 1998b, 2000), the AI has been estimated in a number of different ways (see Appendix F). Because of this, the exact meanings and interpretations differ. In some cases, the AI was based on the observed mean intakes of groups or subpopulations that are maintaining health and nutritional status consistent with an apparent low incidence of inadequacy. In other cases, the AI was derived from the lowest level of intake at which all subjects in an experimental study met the criterion of adequacy; this is different from (and generally lower than) the group mean intake that is consistent with all subjects meeting the criterion of adequacy. The AI was sometimes estimated as an approximation of intake in a group with knowledge of actual requirements of only a few individuals.

The methods of derivation of the AI may differ substantially among nutrients and among life stage groups for the same nutrients; it follows that interpretation and appropriate use of the AI must differ also. In Table 5-1, AIs that represent estimates of desirable group mean intakes are identified. Note that the indicators of adequacy are not always indicators of a classical nutrient deficiency state; in some cases they also include factors that may be directed to decreasing risk of chronic, degenerative diseases. Following, and shown in detail in Appendix F, are some examples of nutrients with an AI and the basis for their derivation:

• Calcium: For infants the AI is a direct estimate of a suitable intake based on average content of human milk for an assumed volume of intake. For adolescents and adults the AI is an approximation of the calcium intake that would be sufficient to maintain desirable rates of calcium retention, as determined from balance studies, factorial estimates of requirements, and limited information on bone mineral content and bone mineral density (IOM, 1997).

• Vitamin D: The AI is a value that appears to be needed to maintain—in a defined group with limited, but uncertain, sun exposure and stores—serum 25-hydroxyvitamin D above the concentration below which vitamin D deficiency rickets or osteomalacia occurs. This concentration is rounded to the nearest 50 IU and then doubled as a safety factor to cover the needs of all people regardless of sun exposure.

• Fluoride: For infants the AI is based on reported group mean intakes; for children and adults the AI is based on factorial esti-

TABLE 5-1 Nutrients with Adequate Intakes (AIs)

Nutrient	Life Stage Group	Group Mean Intake?[a]
Calcium	0–12 mo	Yes
	1–18 y	No
	19–50 y	No
	>51 y	No
	Pregnancy and lactation (all ages)	No
Fluoride	0–12 mo	Yes
	1–18 y	Yes
	19–50 y	Yes
	>51 y	Yes
	Pregnancy and lactation (all ages)	Yes
Magnesium	0–12 mo	Yes
Phosphorus	0–12 mo	Yes
Selenium	0–12 mo	Yes
Biotin	0–12 mo	Yes
	1–18 y	No
	19–50 y	No
	>51 y	No
	Pregnancy and lactation (all ages)	No
Choline	0–12 mo	Yes
	1–18 y	No
	19–50 y	No
	>51 y	No
	Pregnancy and lactation (all ages)	No
Folate	0–12 mo	Yes
Niacin	0–12 mo	Yes
Pantothenic Acid	0–12 mo	Yes
	1–18 y	Yes
	19–50 y	Yes
	>51 y	Yes
	Pregnancy (all ages)	Yes
	Lactation (all ages)	No
Riboflavin	0–12 mo	Yes
Thiamin	0–12 mo	Yes
Vitamin B_6	0–12 mo	Yes
Vitamin B_{12}	0–12 mo	Yes
Vitamin C	0–12 mo	Yes
Vitamin D	0–12 mo	No
	1–18 y	No
	19–50 y	No
	>51 y	No
	Pregnancy and lactation (all ages)	No
Vitamin E	0–12 mo	Yes

[a] See Appendix F for details

mates of suitable group mean intakes. The criterion of adequacy was an intake that would be associated with low occurrence of dental caries.

• Choline: The AI is based on a single experiment in adult men. Choline's potential role in reducing chronic disease risk was considered in developing its AI.

• Biotin: For infants exclusively fed human milk, the AI is based on the biotin content of human milk. This level is extrapolated for all other age groups.

• Pantothenic acid: The AI is based on estimated mean intakes of apparently healthy populations.

COMPARISON OF THE AI, RDA, AND EAR

In general, how does the Adequate Intake (AI) compare with the Estimated Average Requirement (EAR) and the Recommended Dietary Allowance (RDA)?

The amount of evidence suitable for setting the AI is less than that available for setting the EAR and deriving the RDA. When the AI represents a suitable group mean intake, by definition, it is above the (unknown) EAR and generally should be above the (unknown) RDA.

Like the RDAs (which are derived from the EARs), the AIs are levels of nutrient intake that should be associated with a low risk of developing a condition related to a nutrient deficiency or some other negative functional outcome (see Appendix F for details). Intakes at the level of the RDA or AI would not necessarily replete or rehabilitate individuals previously undernourished, nor would they be adequate for persons afflicted by a disease that increased requirements.

LIMITATIONS OF THE AI IN DIETARY ASSESSMENT

Can the Adequate Intake (AI) be used to determine the prevalence of inadequate nutrient intakes in a group?

No.

The AI cannot be used to calculate the prevalence of inadequate nutrient intakes for groups. However, for nutrients with appropriately estimated AIs (see Table 5-1), groups with mean intakes at or above the AI can generally be assumed to have a low prevalence of inadequate intakes (low group risk) for the defined criterion of nutritional status. When mean intakes of groups are below the AI, assumptions cannot be made about inadequacy of intakes (except when intakes are zero, in which case intake is clearly inadequate). Thus, the following statements can be made:

• If the mean intake of a group is at or above the AI, and the variance of intake is similar to the variance of intake in the population originally used to set the AI, the prevalence of inadequate nutrient intakes is likely to be low (although it cannot be estimated) (see Table 5-1 and Appendix F). This evaluation can be used with confidence when the AI is based directly on intakes of healthy populations (as is the case for all AIs except for vitamin D for infants 0 through 12 months of age, for pantothenic acid, and fluoride for children and adults). However, one would have less confidence making this type of evaluation when the AI is not based directly on the intakes of healthy populations.

• If the mean intake is below the AI, the adequacy of the group's intake cannot be determined.

Can the proportion of the population below the AI be used as an indicator of the percentage of the population whose intakes are inadequate?

No.

Because the AI should be above the true Estimated Average Requirement (EAR), any prevalence estimates of nutrient inadequacy calculated by counting individuals with intakes below the AI would be overestimates—potentially major overestimates—of the true prevalence. Thus, although the EAR may be used as a cut-point, *the AI may not be used as a cut-point to estimate the percentage of a population with inadequate intakes.*

Can the relative adequacy of two groups—or of one group at two different times—be assessed by comparing mean intakes with the AI or by comparing the proportion of the groups below the AI?

No.

Because the AI may be above the (unknown) Recommended Dietary Allowance (RDA), mean intakes well below the AI may still have a low prevalence of nutrient inadequacy. It is not possible to know exactly where the mean intake as a percentage of the AI becomes associated with an increased risk of inadequacy. For example, mean intakes at 70 and 90 percent of the AI may have virtually identical very low risks of inadequacy. Therefore, comparisons of this type should be avoided.

Can we calculate back from the AI to a proxy for a nonexistent EAR?

No.

Another potential misuse of the AI is calculating back under the assumption that a proxy for the EAR can be determined. Because the AI is used as a target in counseling individuals—just as the RDA is used as an intake target—there is a strong possibility that the AI will be misused in much the same way as the former RDAs were misused. Some may assume that it is appropriate to use an actual standard deviation of intake or assume a certain coefficient of variation of requirements to calculate back from the AI to a value that might be assumed to be close to the EAR.

Two times the assumed coefficient of variance of requirements (approximately 10 percent) might be subtracted from the AI with the assumption that the resulting number would be a proxy for the requirement. In fact this would only be the case if the AI were set so that only 2 to 3 percent of the population was below the EAR and the requirement was normally distributed (Beaton, 1994). Conceptually this may be the case, but in actuality the AI is derived from a different perspective. In fact, the AI involves significantly more assumptions and judgment, and is set differently for each nutrient. For all of these reasons it is not appropriate to calculate a pseudo EAR from the AI. Such attempts will result in estimates of the prevalence of nutrient inadequacy that are erroneous and usually too high.

SUMMARY

Since the Adequate Intake (AI) is set in different ways for different nutrients and its relationship to the requirement for the nutrient is unknown, it cannot be used to estimate the proportion of the population with inadequate intake.

6

Using the
Tolerable Upper Intake Level
for Nutrient Assessment of
Groups

This chapter briefly describes the concepts underlying the development of the Tolerable Upper Intake Levels (ULs). It also provides guidance on the use of the UL in conjunction with the appropriate usual intake distribution to determine the proportion of individuals in a group who may be potentially at risk of adverse effects due to excessive intake of a nutrient.

THEORY AND DEFINITIONS

Just as quantitative guidelines are needed to help ensure adequacy of nutrient intake, guidelines are needed to help ensure that usual intake levels are not so high that they pose a risk of adverse health effects to an individual or group of individuals. The introduction of the Tolerable Upper Intake Level (UL) is a long overdue contribution to nutritional evaluation. Great effort has been taken in evaluating the published literature relevant to adverse health effects of overconsumption of specific nutrients. The UL is meant to inform the public of risk of excess nutrient intake—*it is not a recommended intake level.*

The UL is determined using a risk assessment model that was developed specifically for nutrients (IOM, 1998a). The model consists of a systematic series of scientific considerations and judgments made by experts knowledgeable in both the nutrients of interest and the practice of risk assessment. These ULs reflect the maximum daily intake levels at which no risk of adverse health effects is expected for almost all individuals in the general population—

including sensitive individuals—when the nutrient is consumed over long periods of time. In other words, the UL is the highest usual intake level of a nutrient that poses no risk of adverse effects. In some cases subpopulations with extreme and distinct vulnerabilities may be at risk with intakes at or even below the UL.[1] The process used to set the UL considers the intakes from all sources: food, water, nutrient supplements, and pharmacological agents, although in some cases the UL may apply only to specific sources.

The dose-response assessment, which concludes with an estimate of the UL, is built upon three toxicological concepts commonly used in assessing the risk of exposures to chemical substances: no-observed-adverse-effect level (NOAEL), lowest-observed-adverse-effect level (LOAEL), and uncertainty factor (UF). These are defined as:

- NOAEL is the highest continuing intake of a nutrient at which no adverse effects have been observed in the individuals or groups studied. In some cases it may be derived from experimental studies in animals. When the available data are not sufficient to reveal the NOAEL, it is necessary to rely on a LOAEL.
- LOAEL is the lowest continuing intake at which an adverse effect has been identified. For some nutrients, it may be derived from experimental studies in animals.
- UFs are applied to the NOAEL, and if necessary to the LOAEL, in an attempt to address both gaps in data and incomplete knowledge regarding the inferences required (e.g., the expected variability in response within the population, or extrapolation from experimental animal to human data).

Scientific judgments are used to assign UFs for each of the specific sources of uncertainty associated with the data available for a nutrient. A composite UF for that nutrient is derived by multiplying the assigned UFs. Larger UFs are applied when animal data are used rather than human data, and in instances where the consequence of overconsumption is serious disease. A UF used to estimate a UL from a LOAEL will be larger than one used if a NOAEL is available. UFs established when this document was written are presented in Table 6-1; they range from 1 (expressing great confidence in the NOAEL) to 36 (reflecting extrapolation from experimental animal to human data and from a LOAEL to a NOAEL and other limitations

---

[1] In this case, the subpopulations are identified and discussed in the individual chapters of the DRI nutrient reports (IOM, 1997, 1998b, 2000).

TABLE 6-1 Tolerable Upper Intake Levels, No-Observed-Adverse-Effect Levels, Lowest-Observed-Adverse-Effect Levels, Uncertainty Factors, and Critical Adverse Effects for Various Nutrients, by Life Stage Group

Nutrient	UL[a]	NOAEL[b]	LOAEL[c]	UF[d]	Critical Adverse Effect
Calcium (mg/d)					Hypercalcemia
Infants (0–12 mo)	ND[e]	—[f]	—	—	and renal
Toddlers (1–3 y)	2,500[g]	—	—	—	insufficiency
Children (4–8 y)	2,500[g]	—	—	—	(milk-alkali
Children (9–13 y)	2,500[g]	—	—	—	syndrome)
Adolescents (14–18 y)	2,500[g]	—	—	—	
Adults (19–70 y)	2,500	—[h]	5,000	2	
Pregnant women	2,500	—	—	—	
Lactating women	2,500	—	—	—	
Older adults (> 70 y)	2,500	—	—	—	
Fluoride (mg/d)					Moderate enamel
Infants (0–6 mo)	0.7	—	0.1[i]	1	fluorosis[j]
Infants (6–12 mo)	0.9	—	0.1[i]	1	
Children (1–3 y)	1.3	—	0.1[i]	1	
Children (4–8 y)	2.2	—	0.1[i]	1	
Children (9–13 y)	10	10	—	1	Skeletal fluorosis
Adolescents (14–18 y)	10	10	—	1	
Adults (19–70 y)	10	10	—	1	
Pregnant women	10	10	—	1	
Lactating women	10	10	—	1	
Older adults (> 70 y)	10	10	—	1	
Magnesium[k] (mg/d)					Diarrhea
Infants (0–12 mo)	ND	—	—	—	
Toddlers (1–3 y)	65[l]	—	—	—	
Children (4–8 y)	110[l]	—	—	—	
Children (9–13 y)	350	—	360	~1	
Adolescents (14–18 y)	350	—	360	~1	
Adults (19–70 y)	350	—	360	~1	
Pregnant women	350	—	—	—	
Lactating women	350	—	—	—	
Older adults (> 70 y)	350	—	360	~1	

continued

TABLE 6-1 Continued

Nutrient	UL^a	$NOAEL^b$	$LOAEL^c$	UF^d	Critical Adverse Effect
Phosphorus (g/d)					Hyperphosphatemia
Infants (0–12 mo)	ND	—	—	—	
Toddlers (1–3 y)	3.0	10.2^m	—	3.3	
Children (4–8 y)	3.0	10.2^m	—	3.3	
Children (9–13 y)	4.0	10.2^m	—	2.5	
Adolescents (14–18 y)	4.0	10.2^m	—	2.5	
Adults (19–70 y)	4.0	10.2	—	2.5	
Pregnant women	3.5	—	—	—	
Lactating women	4.0	10.2	—	2.5	
Older adults (> 70 y)	3.0	10.2	—	3.3	
Selenium (µg/d)					Selenosis
Infants (0–6 mo)	45^n	7 µg/kg	—	1	
Infants (7–12 mo)	60^n	—	—	—	
Children (1–3 y)	$90^{l,n}$	—	—	—	
Children (4–8 y)	$150^{l,n}$	—	—	—	
Children (9–13 y)	$280^{l,n}$	—	—	—	
Adolescents (14–18 y)	400	—	—	—	
Adults (19–70 y)	400	800	—	2	
Pregnant women	400	—	—	—	
Lactating women	400	—	—	—	
Older adults (> 70 y)	400^l	—	—	—	
α-Tocopherol^{k,o}(mg/d)					Increased
Infants (0–12 mo)	ND	—	—	—	tendency to
Children (1–3 y)	$200^{l,n}$	—	—	—	hemorrhage
Children (4–8 y)	$300^{l,n}$	—	—	—	seen in rats
Children (9–13 y)	$600^{l,n}$	—	—	—	
Adolescents (14–18 y)	$800^{l,n}$	—	—	—	
Adults (19–70 y)	$1,000^n$	—	500 mg/kg	36	
Pregnant women	$1,000^n$	—	—	—	
Lactating women	$1,000^n$	—	—	—	
Older adults (> 70 y)	$1,000^n$	—	—	—	
Choline (g/d)					Hypotension
Infants (0–12 mo)	ND	—	—	—	fishy body odor
Children (1–3 y)	$1.0^{l,n}$	—	—	—	
Children (4–8 y)	$1.0^{l,n}$	—	—	—	
Children (9–13 y)	$2.0^{l,n}$	—	—	—	
Adolescents (14 –18 y)	$3.0^{l,n}$	—	—	—	

continued

TABLE 6-1 Continued

Nutrient	UL^a	$NOAEL^b$	$LOAEL^c$	UF^d	Critical Adverse Effect
Adults (19–70 y)	3.5^n	—	7.5	2	
Pregnant women	3.5^n	—	—	—	
Lactating women	3.5^n	—	—	—	
Older adults (> 70 y)	3.5^n	—	—	—	
Folate[k] (µg/d)					Precipitation or
Infants (0–12 mo)	ND	—	—	—	exacerbation of
Toddlers (1–3 y)	$300^{l,n}$	—	—	—	neuropathy in
Children (4–8 y)	$400^{l,n}$	—	—	—	vitamin B_{12}
Children (9–13 y)	$600^{l,n}$	—	—	—	deficient-
Adolescents (14–18 y)	$800^{l,n}$	—	—	—	individuals
Adults (19–70 y)	1,000	—	5,000	5	
Pregnant women	1,000	—	—	—	
Lactating women	1,000	—	—	—	
Older adults (> 70 y)	1,000	—	5,000	5	
Niacin[k] (mg/d)					Vasodilation
Infants (0–12 mo)	ND	—	—	—	(flushing; can
Toddlers (1–3 y)	$10^{l,n}$	—	—	—	involve burning,
Children (4–8 y)	$15^{l,n}$	—	—	—	tingling, and
Children (9–13 y)	$20^{l,n}$	—	—	—	itching sensation,
Adolescents (14–18 y)	$30^{l,n}$	—	—	—	as well as
Adults (19–70 y)	35	—	50	1.5	reddened skin;
Pregnant women	35	—	—	—	occasionally
Lactating women	35	—	—	—	accompanied by
Older adults (> 70 y)	35	—	—	—	pain)
Vitamin B_6 (mg/d)					Sensory
Infants (0–12 mo)	ND	—	—	—	neuropathy
Toddlers (1–3 y)	$30^{l,n}$	—	—	—	
Children (4–8 y)	$40^{l,n}$	—	—	—	
Children (9–13 y)	$60^{l,n}$	—	—	—	
Adolescents (14–18 y)	$80^{l,n}$	—	—	—	
Adults (19–70 y)	100	200	—	2	
Pregnant women	100	—	—	—	
Lactating women	100	—	—	—	
Older adults (> 70 y)	100	—	—	—	

continued

TABLE 6-1 Continued

Nutrient	UL^a	$NOAEL^b$	$LOAEL^c$	UF^d	Critical Adverse Effect
Vitamin C (mg/d)					Osmotic diarrhea
Infants (0–12 mo)	ND	—	—	—	and
Children (1–3 y)	$400^{l,n}$	—	—	—	Gastrointestinal
Children (4–8 y)	$650^{l,n}$	—	—	—	disturbances
Children (9–13 y)	$1,200^{l,n}$	—	—	—	
Adolescents (14–18 y)	$1,800^{l,n}$	—	—	—	
Adults (19–70 y)	2,000	—	3,000	1.5	
Pregnant women	2,000	—	—	—	
Lactating women	2,000	—	—	—	
Older adults (> 70 y)	2,000	—	—	—	
Vitamin D $(\mu g/d)^b$					Hypercalcemia
Infants (0–12 mo)	25	45	—	1.8	
Toddlers (1–3 y)	50^g	—	—	—	
Children (4–8 y)	50^g	—	—	—	
Children (9–13 y)	50^g	—	—	—	
Adolescents (14–18 y)	50^g	—	—	—	
Adults (19–70 y)	50	—	—	—	
Pregnant women	50	60	—	1.2	
Lactating women	50	—	—	—	
Older Adults (> 70 y)	50	—	—	—	

a UL = Tolerable Upper Intake Level: The highest level of daily nutrient intake that is likely to pose no risk of adverse health effects to almost all individuals in the general population. Unless otherwise specified, the UL represents total intake from food, water, and supplements. Because of lack of suitable data, ULs could not be established for thiamin, riboflavin, vitamin B_{12}, pantothenic acid, biotin, or any carotenoids. This signifies a need for data. It does not necessarily signify that people can tolerate chronic intakes of these vitamins at levels exceeding the RDA or AI.

b NOAEL = no-observed-adverse-effect level: the highest intake (or experimental oral dose) of a nutrient at which no adverse effects have been observed in the individuals studied.

c LOAEL = lowest-observed-adverse-effect level: the lowest intake (or experimental oral dose) at which an adverse effect has been identified.

d UF = uncertainty factor: a number that is applied to the NOAEL (or LOAEL) to obtain the UL. The UF incorporates uncertainties associated with extrapolating from the observed data to the general population. UFs established at the time this document was written, some of which are presented in this table, range from 1 (expressing great confidence in the NOAEL) to 36 (reflecting extrapolation from animal to human data and significant limitations in the data).

e ND = not determined or identified. Except for vitamin D, selenium, and fluoride, ULs could not be established for infants. Because of the unique nutritional needs and toxicological sensitivity of infants (0–12 mo), the UL for adults was not adjusted on a body-weight basis to derive a UL for infants (as was done for children and adolescents).

f No data available to identify NOAELs or LOAELs.

g Increased rates of bone formation in toddlers, children, and adolescents suggest the adult UL is appropriate for these age groups.

h A solid value for the NOAEL is not available; however, researchers have observed that daily calcium intakes of 1,500 to 2,400 mg did not result in hypercalcemic syndromes.

i In mg/kg/day.

j Moderate and severe forms of enamel fluorosis are characterized by esthetically objectionable changes in tooth color and surface irregularities. This is regarded as a cosmetic effect rather than a functional adverse effect.

k UL represents intake from supplements, food fortificants, and pharmacological agents only and does not include intake from food and water.

l The UL value for adults was adjusted on a body-weight basis to estimate the UL for children.

m The NOAEL of 10.2 g/d for adults was used to set ULs for all other life stage groups except for pregnant women. The UL for pregnant women was set by decreasing the UL for adults by 15 percent.

n UL values have been rounded.

o The UL for α-tocopherol applies to any form of α-tocopherol.

p As cholecalciferol. 1 μg cholecalciferol = 40 IU vitamin D.

SOURCES: IOM (1997, 1998b, 2000).

in the data). UFs greater than 100 may be required for some nutrients in future evaluations, particularly if data on humans are not available, great uncertainties are found in the dose-response curve, and the adverse effect is not reversible. At a UF of 1, the NOAEL equals the UL.

Information used to establish ULs is summarized in Table 6-1. Readers are referred to the report *Dietary Reference Intakes: A Risk Assessment Model for Establishing Upper Intake Levels for Nutrients* (IOM, 1998a) and the individual nutrient reports (IOM, 1997, 1998b, 2000) for additional information.

EVALUATING THE RISK OF ADVERSE EFFECTS USING THE UL

How to Use ULs

Because the actual risk curve (probability of adverse effect at each level of intake) is unknown, it is not possible to determine the actual risk (likelihood) of adverse health effects for each individual in the general population. Until more research is done in this area, the UL is meant to be used as a guidepost for potential adverse effects and to help ensure that individual intakes do not exceed a safe intake or do so only rarely.

The procedure for applying the UL in assessing the proportion of individuals in a group who are potentially at risk of adverse health effects from excess nutrient intake is similar to the EAR cut-point method described earlier (Chapter 4) for assessing nutrient inadequacy. In this case, one simply determines the proportion of the group with intakes above the UL. However, because the ULs for nutrients are based on different sources of intake, one must be careful to use the appropriate usual intake distribution in the assess-

---

Box 6-1 *Factors to consider when assessing the risk of high intakes:*

- the accuracy of the intake data
- the percentage of the population consistently consuming the nutrient at intake levels in excess of the UL
- the seriousness of the adverse effect
- the extent to which the adverse effect is reversible when intakes are reduced to levels less than the UL.

ment. For some nutrients (e.g., fluoride, phosphorus, vitamin C) the distribution of usual intake would need to include intake from all sources, while for others (e.g., magnesium, folate, niacin, vitamin E) only the distribution of usual supplement intake would be needed.

Figure 6-1 provides a hypothetical example of the relationship between population median intakes and the risk function for intakes at all levels. It can be seen that the percentage of the population at risk would differ depending on the steepness of the risk function. As noted above, however, the risk function (the dose-response curve) for all nutrients is unknown.

Figure 6-2 illustrates a distribution of usual nutrient intakes in a population; the proportion of the population with usual intakes above the UL represents the potential at-risk group. An evaluation of the public health significance of the risk to the population consuming a nutrient in excess of the UL would be required to determine if action was needed.

If no discernible portion of the population consumes the nutrient in excess of the UL, no public health risk should exist. However, if

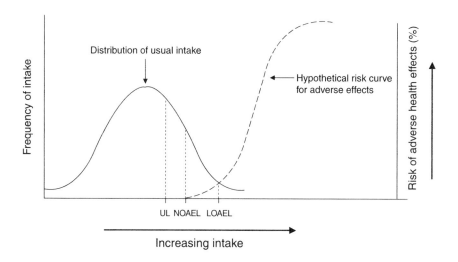

FIGURE 6-1 Hypothetical example of risk of adverse effects compared to population intake. The fraction of the population having usual nutrient intakes above the Tolerable Upper Intake Level (UL) is potentially at risk; the probability of adverse effects increases as nutrient intakes increase above the UL, although the true risk function is not known for most nutrients. NOAEL = no-observed-adverse-effect level, LOAEL = lowest-observed-adverse-effect level.

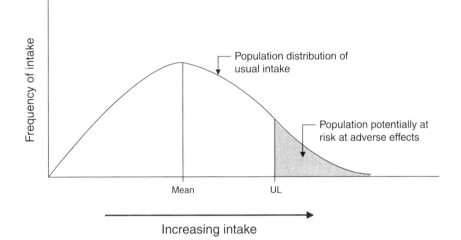

FIGURE 6-2 Population potentially at risk from excessive nutrient intakes. The fraction of the population consistently consuming a nutrient at intake levels in excess of the Tolerable Upper Intake Level (UL) is potentially at risk of adverse health effects. Additional information is necessary to judge the significance of the risk.

some portion of the population has intakes above the UL, a risk may exist and the need to take action to reduce population intakes should be evaluated. For example, the UL for niacin for adults is 35 mg/day. The LOAEL for niacin is 50 mg/day and the uncertainty factor is 1.5 (indicating a good level of confidence in the data). The adverse effect noted is a relatively benign vasodilation causing flushing of the skin that may be accompanied by a burning, itching, or tingling sensation; this effect is readily reversible by a reduction in intake. The UL for vitamin B_6 is 100 mg/day for adults and the NOAEL is 200 mg/day with a UF of 2. The adverse effect observed— sensory neuropathy—is a serious and irreversible condition. Therefore, public health concern over a segment of the population routinely consuming niacin in excess of the UL would not be as great as if a segment of the population were routinely consuming vitamin B_6 in excess of the UL.

Figure 6-3 illustrates a situation in which usual dietary intake from foods represents no discernible risk but the addition of intakes from supplement usage makes a fraction of the population potentially at risk. Figure 6-4 represents the type of analysis that would apply when

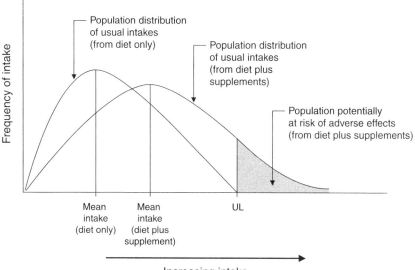

FIGURE 6-3 Effect of including supplement intakes on the population potentially at risk. In this case, nutrient intakes from diet alone are risk-free, but intakes from supplement plus diet put a fraction of the population at risk. The Tolerable Upper Intake Level (UL) here applies to all sources of intake. The significance of the risk is judged by consideration of additional factors.

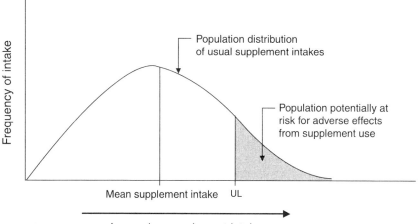

FIGURE 6-4 Risk analysis when the Tolerable Upper Intake Level (UL) applies only to supplements. The significance of the risk is judged by consideration of additional factors.

the data reveal that only supplement usage poses a risk (the UL applies only to the supplement); in this case only the supplement intake distribution requires analysis. For example, for nutrients such as magnesium, folate, niacin, and vitamin E no information exists on adverse effects occurring from the nutrient when consumption is from foods; adverse effects have been seen only when the nutrient was consumed as a supplement, as a fortificant added to food (e.g., folate), or in over-the-counter medications (e.g., magnesium in antacids). In each of these cases the significance of the risk requires consideration of more than the fraction of the population that exceeds the UL. Currently, population usual intake distributions can be estimated, but the shape of the UL risk curve is unknown. When this information is available, however, the probability approach, as described in Chapter 4, can be used to assess the proportion of the population potentially at risk of adverse effects. The underlying assumption is that there is a threshold below which there is negligible risk from overconsumption and above which dose-response curves for toxicological assessment can be linear, exponential, or some other shape.

Although members of the general population should be advised not to routinely exceed the UL, intake above the UL may be appropriate for investigation within well-controlled clinical trials. Clinical trials of doses above the UL should not be discouraged as long as subjects participating in these trials have signed informed consent documents regarding possible adverse effects, and as long as these trials employ appropriate safety monitoring of trial subjects. In addition, the UL is not meant to apply to individuals who are receiving a high dose of a nutrient under medical supervision.

The UL is typically derived to apply to the most sensitive members of the general population. For this reason, many members of the population may regularly consume nutrients at or even somewhat above the UL without experiencing adverse effects. However, because there is no way to establish which individuals are the most sensitive, it is necessary to interpret the UL as applying to all individuals.

Supplement Use

The need for ULs derives largely from regular, self-prescribed use of large amounts of highly fortified foods, regular consumption of a large number of moderately fortified foods, or nonfood sources such as nutritional supplements, or any combination of the three, by significant proportions of the population. Few nutrients are consumed through the food supply in amounts that could cause toxicity.

When this does occur it may be due to composition of the soil, extremely unusual food choices, or errors during food fortification.

The use of nutrient supplements is growing in the United States and Canada, with reports from the Third National Health and Nutrition Examination Survey (NHANES III) suggesting that half the population is using nutritional supplements. Although this information is not sufficiently quantitative for estimations of population intakes, it is known that in some population subgroups nutrient intakes exceed the UL. Supplements should not be treated casually even though excessive intakes appear to be harmless because they are excreted or do not incur a toxic response. It is important to remember that the ULs are based on chronic exposures. The amounts of a nutrient considered toxic upon acute exposure are generally considerably higher than the UL, but have not been established for many nutrients.

SOME FREQUENTLY ASKED QUESTIONS

How serious is the risk of adverse effects for individuals chronically consuming nutrients at levels greater than the Tolerable Upper Intake Level (UL)?

The critical adverse effects used to set the UL are listed in Table 6-1. The dose, the seriousness of the adverse effects, and the extent to which the effects are reversible upon intake reduction should be considered in evaluating the risk of adverse effects.

If the mean intake of a population equals the UL, is there no risk?

A population mean intake at the UL suggests that a large proportion (as much as half) of the population is consuming levels above the UL. This would represent a very serious population risk of adverse effects.

How different are the ULs from doses that would confer acute toxicity?

The ULs are the maximum levels that can be consumed daily on a chronic basis without adverse effects. The ULs will generally be much lower than the levels that are necessary to produce adverse effects after a single exposure. Few evaluations of the acute toxic intake of nutrients have been made.

How close are the Recommended Dietary Allowances (RDAs) and ULs?

There is no standard or definable mathematical relationship between the RDA and the UL. For some nutrients, the two values are widely separated (for example, the RDA for vitamin B_6 for adult women is 1.3 mg/day, whereas the UL is 100 mg/day). In some cases the two standards cannot be compared directly because the UL is to be applied only to sources of the nutrient that are not naturally in foods (e.g., the UL for magnesium is only for intake from supplements).

Will we find out in a few years that the RDA and Adequate Intake (AI) are too low and that higher nutrient intakes are better to prevent specific diseases such as cancer?

As our ability to study the chronic effects of various levels of nutrient intakes on humans improves, our knowledge of the relationships between single nutrients and disease prevention will improve. As a result, suggested desirable intake may increase or decrease. Higher nutrient intakes may not be found to be better. In some clinical intervention trials, high doses of β-carotene being studied for cancer prevention were reported to actually increase the risk of lung cancer in long-term current smokers. This demonstrates that it is difficult to speculate about even the direction of an effect when an individual consumes high doses of a nutrient (those that greatly exceed the amounts found in foods).

7

Specific Applications: Assessing Nutrient Intakes of Groups Using the Dietary Reference Intakes

This chapter focuses on specific applications of the Dietary Reference Intakes (DRIs) to assess the nutrient adequacy of groups, in particular describing and evaluating dietary survey data. The methodological approaches described in Chapters 4, 5, and 6 are applied to some of the specific uses reported in Chapter 2. (Chapter 3 presents an application for assessing the nutrient adequacy of individual diets.) A subsequent report will examine applications of the DRIs for planning nutrient intakes of groups and individuals, which includes many of the other uses presented in Chapter 2.

INTRODUCTION

Assessment of the apparent nutrient adequacy of groups typically has used the former Recommended Dietary Allowances (RDAs) and Recommended Nutrient Intakes (RNIs) because these were the primary dietary standards that were available. In many instances, however, the former RDAs and RNIs were used inappropriately in dietary assessment applications (e.g., RDAs used for dietary assessment of groups, with some arbitrary percentage of the RDA used as a cut-point for determining nutrient adequacy of a group).

The applications considered in this chapter are designed to analyze information about the distribution of average daily intakes over time, referred to as usual nutrient intakes. Typically, though, survey data on nutrient intakes of the same individual are only available for one or two days; sometimes two or more nonconsecutive days of dietary recall data are available for a subsample of individuals, with one day of recall data available for the remainder of the sample.

Thus, to conduct evaluations of dietary survey data, it is usually necessary first to adjust the intake distributions based on at least two nonconsecutive days of dietary recalls to obtain the usual nutrient intake distribution. If these adjustments are not made, outcome variables that rely on any measure other than the group's mean intake are biased (Carriquiry et al., 1997; Nusser et al., 1996). For example, the percentage of individuals in a group with intakes less than a specified cutoff level would be biased (either over- or underestimated) if determined from unadjusted data on nutrient intakes. See Chapter 4 for methods to adjust intake distributions.

APPLICATION 1: DESCRIBING DIETARY SURVEY DATA

What are the characteristics of the distributions of usual nutrient intake? How variable are usual intakes?

Data available: 24-hour dietary recall data on a nationally representative sample of individuals, with two or more nonconsecutive days of data collected for at least a subsample of individuals.

This discussion assumes that dietary recall data are available from a nationally representative sample of individuals and have been used to estimate the usual nutrient intakes of the population from food and supplements.

The following summary descriptive measures could be examined: mean, median, and other percentiles of the usual nutrient intake distribution. An example of appropriate descriptive statistics is given in Table 7-1.

Many researchers have expressed intakes as a percentage of the Recommended Dietary Allowance (RDA) primarily to aid the interpretation of descriptive statistics across life stage and gender groups that have different requirements. Although expressing mean intake as a percentage of the RDA is not incorrect, it is easily misinterpreted. These statistics cannot be used to assess nutrient adequacy.

TABLE 7-1 Describing Nutrient Intakes of Children 4 through 8 Years of Age—Characteristics of Usual Nutrient Intake

| Nutrient | Unit | Nutrient Reference Intake[a] | | | Usual Nutrient Intake* | |
		EAR	RDA	AI	Mean Intake	Median Intake
Calcium	mg/d	NA[b]	NA	800	838	808
Phosphorus	mg/d	405	500	NA	1,088	1,059
Magnesium	mg/d	110	130	NA	212	205
Thiamin	mg/d	0.5	0.6	NA	1.44	1.40
Riboflavin	mg/d	0.5	0.6	NA	1.91	1.84
Niacin	mg/d	6	8	NA	17.6	17.1
Vitamin B_6	mg/d	0.5	0.6	NA	1.53	1.48
Folate[c]	μg/d	160	200	NA	232	221
Vitamin B_{12}	μg/d	1.0	1.2	NA	3.83	3.62
Vitamin C	mg/d	22	25	NA	96.5	90.0
Vitamin E[d,e]	mg/d	6	7	NA	5.8	5.6
Selenium[e]	μg/d	23	30	NA	86.8	85.0

[a] EAR = Estimated Average Requirement; RDA = Recommended Dietary Allowance; AI = Adequate Intake.

[b] NA = not applicable.

[c] The EAR and RDA for folate are expressed as μg dietary folate equivalents (DFE). However, insufficient information was available to convert intake data from the Continuing Survey of Food Intakes by Individuals to DFEs, thus for this example, folate intake is expressed in micrograms.

[d] Mean and median intake expressed as mg of α-tocopherol.

[e] Dietary intake data for selenium and vitamin E are from the Third National Health and Nutrition Examination Survey, 1988–1994.

SOURCE: 1994–1996 Continuing Survey of Food Intakes by Individuals.

*NOTE: Does not include intake from supplements.

APPLICATION 2: ASSESSING THE PREVALENCE OF INADEQUATE OR EXCESSIVE INTAKE

What proportion of the population has inadequate nutrient intake? What proportion of the population is at risk of excessive nutrient intake?

Data available: 24-hour dietary recall data on a nationally representative sample of individuals, with two or more nonconsecutive days of data collected for at least a subsample of individuals.

Comparing Usual Intakes with the EAR and the UL

Table 7-2 is an example of an evaluation of the intakes of children 4 through 8 years of age. Under certain assumptions an effective estimate of the prevalence of inadequate intake is the percentage of a group with usual nutrient intake less than the Estimated Average Requirement (EAR). Dietary Reference Intakes (DRIs) have not yet

TABLE 7-2 Assessing Nutrient Intakes of Children 4 through 8 Years of Age—What Proportion Has Inadequate Intake? What Proportion Is Potentially at Risk of Excessive Intake?

Nutrient	Unit	EAR[a]	Percentage Less than the EAR	UL[b]	Percentage Greater than the UL
Calcium	mg/d	NA[c]	NA	2,500	<1
Phosphorus	mg/d	405	<1	3,000	<1
Magnesium	mg/d	110	5	110[d]	UK[e]
Thiamin	mg/d	0.5	<1	NA	NA
Riboflavin	mg/d	0.5	<1	NA	NA
Niacin	mg/d	6	<1	15	UK
Vitamin B_6	mg/d	0.5	<1	40	<1
Folate[f]	µg/d	160	35	400	UK
Vitamin B_{12}	µg/d	1.0	<1	NA	NA
Vitamin C	mg/d	22	<1	650	<1
Vitamin E[g,h]	mg/d	6	60[i]	300[j]	UK
Selenium[h]	µg/d	23	<1	150	<1

[a] EAR=Estimated Average Requirement.
[b] UL=Tolerable Upper Intake Level.
[c] NA = not applicable.
[d] UL for magnesium applies to supplements only, not diet plus supplement.
[e] UK = Unknown because the UL applies only to intakes from supplements (magnesium) or from supplemental and fortification sources (niacin, folate, and vitamin E).
[f] The EAR and RDA for folate are expressed as µg dietary folate equivalents (DFE). However, insufficient information was available to convert intake data from the Continuing Survey of Food Intakes by Individuals to DFEs, thus for this example, folate intake is expressed in µg. Intake data were collected prior to folate fortification of grain products and thus underestimate current folate intake.
[g] The EAR is expressed in mg of α-tocopherol.
[h] Dietary intake data for selenium and vitamin E is from the Third National Health and Nutrition Examination Survey, 1988–1994.
[i] Accurate measures of vitamin E intake are difficult to obtain due to underreporting of fat intake; it is likely that the percent less than the EAR is an overestimate (IOM, 2000).
[j] Applies to any form of supplemental α-tocopherol.
SOURCE: 1994–1996 Continuing Survey of Food Intakes by Individuals.

been established for all nutrients, and some nutrients have Adequate Intakes (AIs) rather than EARs. As a result the only nutrients to which the probability approach or the EAR cut-point method (described in Chapter 4) can be applied to assess adequacy in this example are vitamin B_6, vitamin B_{12}, vitamin C, vitamin E, folate, niacin, riboflavin, thiamin, magnesium, phosphorus, and selenium. Additional nutrients will be added as DRIs are developed for them.

   To estimate the proportion of the population potentially at risk from excessive intake, the percentage of the group with usual nutrient intake exceeding the Tolerable Upper Intake Level (UL) is determined (see Chapter 6). Again, because ULs have not yet been established for all nutrients, the only nutrients for which the proportion at risk for excessive intake can be estimated are niacin, vitamin B_6, folate, choline, vitamin C, vitamin D, vitamin E, calcium, phosphorus, magnesium, fluoride, and selenium. Additional nutrients will also be added to this list as DRIs are developed for them. It should be noted however, that even though EARs or ULs are currently available for some nutrients (e.g., vitamin D, fluoride, and choline), assessment of adequacy or potential risk of excess is not possible because these nutrients are not included in the national intake surveys.

Common Mistakes in Evaluating Dietary Survey Data

   Some of the most common mistakes in evaluating dietary survey data arise from inappropriate conclusions drawn from comparing mean nutrient intakes with Recommended Dietary Allowances (RDAs). When mean nutrient intake exceeds the RDA, researchers often conclude—inappropriately—that diets meet or even exceed recommended nutritional standards. At one time, when the RDA was defined as the average intake of a population, this mistake was understandable. However, the current definition of the RDA (and the definition implied in the last two revisions [NRC, 1980, 1989]) specifically defines the RDA as a goal for the individual. In fact, as discussed in Chapter 4, because the variance of usual intake typically exceeds the variance of nutrient requirement for most nutrients, the mean usual nutrient intake of a group must exceed the RDA to have a low prevalence of inadequate intakes. Even if mean usual nutrient intake equals or exceeds the RDA, a significant proportion of the population may have inadequate nutrient intake. This is clearly shown in Tables 7-1 and 7-2, where both the mean and median of usual intake of folate exceed the RDA, yet approximately 35 percent of children 4 through 8 years of age are estimated to have usual intake less than the requirement.

Mean or median intakes of nutrients with EARs seldom, if ever, can be used to assess adequacy or excessive intake of group diets. *The prevalence of inadequacy depends on the shape and variation of the usual intake distribution, not on mean intake.* For food energy, however, mean intake relative to the EAR is a possible measure to use in assessing the adequacy of group diets. Because there is a high correlation between energy intake and energy expenditure (requirement), median intake of food energy should be close to the requirement for there to be low risk of inadequate or excessive intake.

Caution also is necessary when interpreting descriptive statistics for nutrients with an AI. When mean usual intake of a group exceeds the AI the expected prevalence of inadequate intake is low. When mean usual nutrient intake of a group is less than the AI, however, nothing can be inferred about the probability of inadequacy (see Chapter 5).

In short, comparing mean intake either to the EAR or RDA or simply looking at mean intake levels should not be used to assess or imply relative nutrient adequacy.

APPLICATION 3: EVALUATING DIFFERENCES IN INTAKE

Do different subgroups of the population (food stamp participants and nonparticipants, for example) differ in their mean nutrient intakes?

  • *What are the characteristics of the usual nutrient intake distribution for different population subgroups? Do population subgroups have different distributions of usual nutrient intake?*
  • *Do population subgroups differ in the proportion with inadequate nutrient intake?*
  • *Do population subgroups differ in the proportion at risk of excessive nutrient intake?*

Research studies often focus either on differences in nutrient intake for population subgroups or on the relationship between certain factors and nutrient intakes. Such studies are simply extensions of the dietary survey applications discussed above. They typically use both descriptive and multiple regression analyses to examine differences in nutrient intakes across population subgroups. Descriptive analyses compare differences across subgroups in means, medians, and percentages with intake less than the Estimated Average Requirement (EAR) or exceeding the Tolerable Upper Intake Level (UL). Multiple regression analyses use individual data on nutrient intakes to estimate the effects of various factors on nutrient intake. The results can be used to present regression-adjusted differences in measures among the subgroups.

As an example of this application, consider an evaluation of the Food Stamp Program (FSP) that involves estimating the relationship between FSP participation and nutrient intakes. In this application, 24-hour dietary recall data are available on a nationally representative sample of individuals eligible for the FSP. This sample includes both FSP participants and low-income nonparticipants.

Descriptive Analyses of Nutrient Intakes

Descriptive analyses would examine the mean, median, and other selected percentiles of the usual nutrient intake distribution.

Statistical tests can be conducted to determine whether FSP participation is associated with differences in nutrient intake. In this case, if comparison of the means is all that is wanted (although of limited value), no adjustments for usual intake are necessary and a t-test can be used. However, before performing these tests, it is important to consider survey weights and survey design effects. If sampled individuals have different survey weights attached to them (see Chapter 4), the mean and the standard error of the mean need to be computed using these weights. If the survey design is clustered, the variance can be artificially reduced and thus needs to be adjusted. Various software programs can be used for this purpose.[1]

However, if interest is on information at the tails of the distributions (i.e., percentiles), adjustment of the intake distributions to obtain the usual nutrient intake distributions from the observed nutrient intake distributions is needed to more accurately reflect

---

[1] Software programs exist to calculate t-tests of the differences between means when sample individuals have different survey weights and the survey has a cluster design. Software programs that can be used include SUDAAN (Software for the Statistical Analysis of Correlated Data, Research Triangle Institute, 3040 Cornwallis Road, PO Box 12194, Research Triangle Park, NC 27709-2194), WESVAR (Westat Variance, Westat, 1650 Research Blvd., Rockville, MD 20850), and PC-CARP (Personal Computer Cluster Analysis and Regression Program, Statistical Laboratory, Iowa State University, Ames, IA 50011-1210).

the individual-to-individual variation in intake. For example, one might wish to determine whether the proportion of individuals with inadequate intakes is different among FSP participants and low-income nonparticipants.

To describe differences in the prevalence of apparently inadequate nutrient intakes between subgroups, the percentages of FSP participants and low-income nonparticipants with usual nutrient intake less than the EAR (for nutrients with an EAR) should be calculated and compared. Similarly, to describe differences in the percentage potentially at risk from excessive nutrient intakes by subgroup, the percentages of FSP participants and low-income nonparticipants with usual nutrient intake greater than the UL (for nutrients with a UL) should be calculated and compared. Tests such as t-tests can then be conducted to determine whether these differences are statistically significant.

Multiple Regression Analyses of Nutrient Intake

One important objective of multiple regression analysis is to correct the simple difference in group mean intake discussed above for other differences between subgroups. For example, suppose FSP participants and low-income nonparticipants differ in their characteristics (such as household income or family size) and that these differences also affect nutrient intake. Multiple regression analyses (straightforward analyses of covariance) can adjust the simple difference in mean nutrient intake between FSP participants and nonparticipants for differences attributed to household income and family size. The results of these analyses can be used to calculate regression-adjusted differences in nutrient intake for different population subgroups.

In multiple regression analysis, the dependent variable refers to an individual, not to a group. As noted previously, individual nutrient intake observed on one day is not the same as usual nutrient intake for that individual. Although adjustments can be made to the intake distribution of a group to estimate the usual intake distribution (see Chapter 4), adjustments cannot usually be made to individual values to estimate usual individual intake. The discussion below focuses on using observed nutrient intake data for individuals to define dependent variables for multiple regression analyses, how to interpret the results from the regression analyses, and how to use the results of these analyses to assess differences in nutrient adequacy across subgroups.

Regression-Adjusted Differences in Mean Nutrient Intakes

For a multiple regression analysis of nutrient intakes, the dependent variable is usually the observed individual nutrient intake. In the context of the FSP, the dependent variable would be observed nutrient intakes while predictor variables might include—in addition to food stamp participation—household income, family size, education, region of residence, and other important characteristics influencing nutrient intake. This type of multiple regression analysis typically produces a set of regression coefficients and their standard deviations. On the basis of the estimated coefficient for FSP participation, regression-adjusted differences in mean nutrient intake can be calculated between FSP participants and low-income nonparticipants, controlling for other differences between participants and nonparticipants that may also influence nutrient intake. In addition, just as the mean of observed nutrient intake is an unbiased estimate of mean usual nutrient intake, these regression-adjusted differences in mean observed intakes are unbiased estimates of regression-adjusted mean usual nutrient intake.

Multiple regression analysis of nutrient intakes has been used to assess the relationship between program participation and nutrient intakes in FSP eligible individuals (Gordon et al., 1995; Oliveira and Gunderson, 2000; Rose et al., 1998). Specifically, the regression-adjusted differences in mean intake between program participants and a comparison group of nonparticipants were interpreted, with certain caveats, as the estimated effects of program participation. However, as noted previously, mean intakes cannot be used to assess nutrient adequacy. Similarly, differences in mean intakes between subgroups cannot be used to draw conclusions about the effects of program participation on nutrient adequacy. They can be used only to make inferences about differences in mean intakes between program participants and nonparticipants. The approach described below provides a method of estimating the effect of FSP participation on nutrient adequacy.

Comparison of the Prevalence of Inadequate Nutrient Intakes

As discussed above, multiple regression analysis can be used to estimate differences in mean intakes between two subgroups such as FSP participants and eligible nonparticipants, while controlling for other factors that affect nutrient intake. A more difficult research question, however, is testing the difference between subgroups in the prevalence of apparent nutrient inadequacy, *after controlling for other factors that affect nutrient intake.* This analysis involves comparing changes to the tail of the intake distributions. In the context of the FSP, the question is whether the proportion of individuals with usual intakes below the EAR is different between FSP participants and nonparticipants, after controlling for other factors that affect nutrient intake.

A proposed approach that enables users to control for effects of potentially confounding variables through regression analysis is outlined below, using the FSP as an example. The required data include:

- *one day of intake data for each person*
- *two independent days of intake for at least a subsample of each group (however, one day of intake data on each individual suffices if only the difference in group mean intake is of interest)*
- *each person's values for each of the potentially confounding variables (e.g., income, education, age, etc.), or at least a reliably imputed value, as well as an indicator for FSP participation status (e.g., participant, nonparticipant).*

Step 1. First, a regression equation is fitted to the observed intake data. Variables in the regression model would include FSP participation (coded as 0 or 1) and any other variables thought to affect intakes. For example, if age were the only other variable considered relevant, the equation would be:

Observed intake (Y) = constant + B_1(age) + B_2(FSP participation) + error.

The fitted regression equation would contain estimated values for the constant and the regression coefficients for FSP participation and for any other variable that was included in the model. These estimated values are denoted as b_1, b_2, b_3, etc.

Step 2. Given the estimated regression coefficients from the first step, a standard predicted intake value is generated for each individual by inserting the values of the covariates for the individual, *appropriately centered*, into the fitted regression equation. The modifier "standard" is used because in this step, one standardizes individual intakes to those that would be observed if everyone in the sample had been, for example, the same age and had the same income. Suppose that the sample consisted of all women aged 20 to 50. A good centering or standardizing age would be 35, the midpoint of the sample age range. This step therefore, standardizes all intakes to values that would have been observed had all sampled individuals differed *only* in the FSP participation status. If age were the only other covariate, the standardized predicted intakes would be calculated as:

Standardized predicted intake = observed intake $(Y) - b_1(\text{age} - 35)$,

where b_1 is the estimated regression coefficient associated with age.

If age is the only covariate (other than FSP participation) believed to be associated with intake, the standard predicted intakes above would correspond to intake values adjusted to a standard age (in this case 35). In essence, step 2 removes the effect of the covariates other than FSP participation on intakes. If the effect of age is to increase intake (i.e., if b_1 is positive), then the standard predicted intakes for individuals who are younger than 35 will be larger than the observed intake for those individuals. On the other hand, the standard predicted intakes for individuals who are older than 35 will be smaller than the intakes observed.

Step 3. Next, the effect of day-to-day variability is removed from the standardized predicted intakes to produce an adjusted usual intake distribution. This step, described previously in Chapter 4, would be done separately for the two groups. Once an adjusted usual intake distribution has been obtained (standardized, for example, to age 35) for each group of individuals, the proportion of each group with intakes below the EAR can then be determined and compared using a simple t-test.

It is important to note that:

• The estimates of prevalence of inadequacy in each of the two groups obtained using the adjusted standardized intakes will be biased, and perhaps severely so. This is because the adjusted standardized intakes have a variability that is too small. When using the standardized intakes in the adjustment procedure, one proceeds as if the regression coefficient b_1 was a known, fixed value. In reality, b_1 is an estimate, and as such has a variance that is not "added" to the variance of observed intakes. However, the *difference between the prevalence estimates for the two groups will still be approximately unbiased*, as long as the distribution of ages among the two participation groups is approximately similar, or as long as individuals in one group tend to be younger than individuals in the other group. If, however, all individuals in one group have ages clustered around the centering age value, while all individuals in the other group have ages that are either much lower or much higher than the centering value, then the adjustment above will lead to biased inferences about the effect of FSP participation on the prevalence of inadequacy.

• Only one covariate has been included in this example. The approach above extends naturally to the case of more than one covariate, and the same centering principle would hold. If, for example, income was a second covariate and if the range of incomes in the sample went from $10,000 to $40,000, then the appropriate centering value for income would be the midpoint ($40,000 - $10,000)/2 + $10,000 = $25,000. In this case, one would be adjusting observed intakes to look like the intakes that would have been observed if all individuals had been 35 years of age and earned $25,000.

• The adjustment above relies on the ability to accurately specify a regression model for intake. The model needs to contain all covariates thought to be associated with intake, particularly if they are also thought to be correlated with FSP participation. The estimated regression coefficients will have better statistical properties when intakes are approximately normally distributed.

The hypothetical example below (see also Table 7-3) illustrates the first four steps of this approach to assess whether FSP participation affects the mean intake of the group or the prevalence of inadequacy of nutrient A. In this example, it is suspected that age may influence intake of nutrient A and may also be associated with FSP participation. For each of a large group of individuals, 2 days of intake data are available, and the age of each individual is known. Some are FSP participants (FSP = 1) and others are not (FSP = 0). The overall group mean intake of nutrient A is 772 units. Table 7-3 shows data for six of these individuals.

Step 1. In the first step, a regression model is fitted to the intake data (column 4 of the table). The resulting prediction equation is:

$$\text{Observed intake} = -9 + 21.7 \times \text{age} + 68.7 \times \text{FSP}$$

Step 2. Next, standard predicted intakes are calculated for each individual for each day of intake. The regression coefficient associated with age generated from the intake data is used, but the coefficient for FSP participation and the intercept are not included. The

TABLE 7-3 Data for Six Individuals from a (Hypothetical) Large Survey of Food Stamp Program (FSP) Participants and Nonparticipants

Individual	FSP Participant (1=yes; 0=no)	Age	Observed Intake[a]	Standardized Predicted Intake[b]
1	1	23	558	819
			657	918
2	1	39	825	738
			1,024	937
3	1	36	871	850
			964	943
151	0	44	995	800
			922	726
152	0	37	799	755
			740	696
153	0	40	890	781
			874	765

[a] These values represent the actual intakes for each individual on the 2 days for which diet records were kept.
[b] Standardized predicted intake is calculated as: observed intake (Y) − b_1(age − 35). The value for b_1 is 21.7 in this example.

centering value chosen for age is 35, the midpoint of the range of ages among individuals. Thus, the equation used is:

Standardized predicted intake = observed intake (Y) − 21.7 × (age − 35),

these intakes are shown in the last column of the table.

Step 3. Age-standardized intakes are then used in transformations to remove the effect of day-to-day variability, leading to age-standardized usual intake distributions for FSP participants and FSP nonparticipants (see Chapter 4). Note that these distributions will have the incorrect spread relative to the distribution of usual intakes that would be obtained if individuals had not been standardized to have the same age.

Step 4. Finally, the proportion of individuals with intakes below the EAR in each age-adjusted usual intake distribution can be compared to determine whether FSP participation affects the prevalence of nutrient inadequacy. The actual estimates of inadequacy in each group are meaningless; only the difference between the two prevalence estimates is approximately unbiased.

Cautions Regarding the Use of Binary Variables for Inadequacy

In an analysis of the probability of inadequacy, researchers might be tempted to determine differences in nutrient adequacy between two groups by obtaining an estimate of each individual's usual intake (perhaps by using the observed mean intake as the estimate) and then determining whether the individual is consuming adequate amounts of the nutrient by comparing the intake to the EAR. In this way, a categorical variable with two values (0 for inadequate, 1 for adequate) can be created and used as a response variable in a regression.

Dependent variables should not be binary variables for inadequacy, defined on the basis of nutrient intake below the EAR or below any other threshold value. This is because an individual's true requirement is unknown. Individuals whose usual nutrient intake is below the EAR may still be meeting their own nutrient requirement; while individuals whose usual nutrient intake is above the EAR may not be satisfying their individual nutrient requirement. As a result, a binary variable denoting whether an individual's usual nutrient intake is less than the EAR will misclassify some individuals.[2]

A second problem associated with using a binary variable to denote nutrient inadequacy is that observed nutrient intake for an individual differs from usual nutrient intake. Therefore, some individuals will be classified as below the EAR on the basis of observed nutrient intake although their usual nutrient intake would put them above the EAR, and vice versa. In general, because of underreporting, using observed nutrient intake data overstates the proportion of individuals with usual nutrient intakes less than the EAR.

As a result of both of these considerations, a logistic regression for multivariate analysis in which the response variable is a binary variable constructed by comparing the individual's intake to the EAR will lead to biased estimates of the effects of the covariates on the probability of inadequacy.

---

[2] For a group, the percentage with usual intake less than the EAR is a good estimate of the proportion with inadequate usual nutrient intake because those individuals who are misclassified cancel each other out. That is, the individuals with usual nutrient intake less than the EAR who are still meeting their requirement are offset by the individuals with usual nutrient intake above the EAR who are not meeting their requirement (triangles A and B of Figure 4-8).

SUMMARY

Table 7-4 summarizes these applications of the Dietary Reference Intakes (DRIs) to assess nutrient intakes of groups. Answers to many of the descriptive questions—such as those regarding the characteristics of the distribution of usual nutrient intake and differences in mean nutrient intakes between population subgroups—do not depend on the DRIs. However, determining the proportion of a group with inadequate usual nutrient intake is only possible for nutrients with Estimated Average Requirements (EARs). Determining the proportion of a group potentially at risk of adverse effects due to excessive usual nutrient intake is only possible for nutrients with Tolerable Upper Intake Levels (ULs). DRIs have not yet been established for many important nutrients and either an EAR or a UL has not yet been determined for others. An important issue, therefore, is what to do until the DRIs are established for these other nutrients. Descriptive applications (such as the example in Table 7-1) might combine information for nutrients with DRIs along with nutrients for which only the older Recommended Dietary Allowances (RDAs) or Recommended Nutrient Intakes (RNIs) are available. However, for evaluation measures (such as the example summarized in Table 7-2), nutrients or food components which do not yet have EARs and ULs under the DRI process should be omitted from applications that assess the prevalence of inadequate intakes or those at potential risk of adverse effects due to excessive intakes.

TABLE 7-4 Applications: Evaluating Dietary Survey Data

Measures	Nutrients

What are the characteristics of the distribution of usual nutrient intake?

Measures	Nutrients
Mean nutrient intake Median usual nutrient intake Percentiles of usual nutrient intake distribution	All nutrients under consideration

What proportion of the population has inadequate usual nutrient intake?

Measures	Nutrients

Percentage with usual intake less
   than the Estimated Average
   Requirement (EAR)
	Vitamins: thiamin, riboflavin, niacin, B_6,
	   folate, B_{12}, C, E
	Elements: phosphorus, magnesium,
	   selenium

What proportion of the population is at potential risk of adverse effects?

Measures	Nutrients

Percentage with usual intake greater
   than the Tolerable Upper Intake
   Level (UL)
	Vitamins: niacin, B_6, folate, choline,
	   C, D, E
	Elements: calcium, phosphorus,
	   magnesium, fluoride, selenium

Are there differences in nutrient intakes and differences in nutrient adequacy for different subgroups of the population?

Measures	Nutrients

Mean nutrient intake for subgroups
Median usual nutrient intake for
   subgroups
Percentiles of the usual nutrient
   intake distribution for subgroups
	All nutrients under consideration

Percentage with usual intake less
   than the EAR for subgroups
	Vitamins: thiamin, riboflavin, niacin, B_6,
	   folate, B_{12}, C, E
	Elements: phosphorus, magnesium,
	   selenium

Percentage with usual intake greater
   than UL for subgroups
	Vitamins: niacin, B_6, folate, choline,
	   C, D, E
	Elements: calcium, phosphorus,
	   magnesium, fluoride, selenium

Comments

Mean nutrient intake should not be used to assess nutrient adequacy.

This measure is not appropriate for food energy, given the correlation between intake and requirement.

This measure is not appropriate for nutrients for which an EAR has not been set.

This measure is not appropriate for nutrients for which a UL has not been set.

Conduct multiple regression analyses of nutrient intakes; compare regression-adjusted mean intake for the different subgroups.

Regression-adjusted mean nutrient intake should not be used to assess nutrient adequacy.

Statistical tests of significance can be used to determine whether the differences across subgroups in percentages less than the EAR are statistically significant.

This measure is not appropriate for food energy because of the correlation between intake and requirement.

This measure is not appropriate for nutrients for which an EAR has not been set.

Statistical tests of significance can be used to determine whether the differences across subgroups in percentages greater than the UL are statistically significant.

This measure is not appropriate for nutrients for which a UL has not been set.

IV

Fine-Tuning Dietary Assessment Using the DRIs

In Part IV, the report examines issues that may affect the dietary assessment methods that are described in Parts II and III and highlights areas of research that need attention.

A brief description of ways to increase the accuracy in the measurement of intakes and requirements, and the importance of representative sampling techniques are highlighted in Chapter 8. Chapter 9 provides recommendations for research needed to improve and refine nutrient assessments.

8

Minimizing Potential Errors in Assessing Group and Individual Intakes

This chapter presents information on ways to minimize errors in dietary assessments, including tailoring the Dietary Reference Intakes (DRIs) to the specific group or individual, ensuring that the intake data have the highest accuracy feasible, minimizing sampling errors when collecting intake data on groups, and determining standard deviations of prevalence estimates.

Dietary assessments involve comparing nutrient intakes of individuals or groups with the DRIs. Thus, there are two primary areas where potential measurement errors can influence assessment results: (1) determining nutrient requirements; and (2) measuring dietary intake, including using appropriate sampling strategies, and accurate nutrient composition for foods consumed.

Intake data need to be collected with the most accurate techniques available, with cost and feasibility of evaluations taken into account. Furthermore, the assessment must use appropriate DRIs, and consider the age, gender, physiological status, and other relevant characteristics (e.g., smoking status) of the individual or group being assessed. If estimates of intakes or requirements (or upper limits) are incorrect, the assessment of inadequate or excess nutrient intakes for the individual or the group will also be incorrect.

TAILORING REQUIREMENTS FOR SPECIFIC GROUPS AND INDIVIDUALS

The Dietary Reference Intakes (DRIs) can be adjusted to be more appropriate for specific individuals or groups. For example, adjust-

147

ments might be made for body size, energy intake, or physiological status. However, such adjustments are usually not necessary since the DRIs are assumed to apply to all healthy individuals in the specified life stage and gender group.

Are there situations when adjustments to the Estimated Average Requirement (EAR), and thus the RDA, should be made for certain individuals to ensure that they are at little or no risk of nutrient inadequacy?

In most cases, adjustments are not likely to be required because the EAR already accounts for normal individual variability. However, adjustments may be warranted for individuals who have unusually high or low body weight, experience physiological changes at unusual ages, experience unusual physiological changes, or have unusually high energy requirements. These situations are discussed below.

Body Weight

When nutrient recommendations are established in relation to body weight, the weight of a reference individual is often used to derive DRIs. (See Appendix A for reference weights used in developing the DRIs.) For example, the RDA for protein has traditionally been related to body weight and in the 10th edition of the RDAs (NRC, 1989) the RDA for protein was set at 0.8 g of protein per kg body weight. Summary tables list RDAs of 63 and 50 g/day of protein, respectively, for reference adult men and women weighing 79 and 63 kg (NRC, 1989). Recommendations for individuals above or below these reference weights would be modified accordingly. For example, the RDA for individuals weighing 45 and 100 kg would be 36 and 80 g/day of protein, respectively. When this adjustment is made the individuals are assumed to have relatively normal body composition because protein requirements are related more strongly to lean body mass than to adipose tissue mass. Thus, a protein intake of 160 g/day would not be recommended for an obese individual weighing 200 kg. None of the DRIs established at the time this report went to press have been expressed in relation to body weight.

Age and Physiological Stage

For some nutrients, requirements change across the lifespan in association with physiological changes that are assumed to occur at various average ages. For example, the AI for vitamin D is higher for adults older than 50 years than for those younger than 50 years, and the recommendation for vitamin B_{12} is that individuals older than 50 years obtain most of their vitamin B_{12} from fortified foods or supplements. For these nutrients, the changes in recommendations are associated with age-related changes in vitamin D metabolism and in gastric acidity, respectively. These changes do not occur abruptly at age 50 and it could reasonably be suggested that average dietary requirements would be increased at the upper end of the 51- through 70-year age range.

In other situations the physiological changes that result in different requirements occur over a shorter time or can be identified by individuals. An example would be iron requirements of women. The requirements for women ages 31 through 50 years are intended to cover losses associated with menstruation whereas for women older than 50 years it is assumed that menopause has occurred. Onset of menopause, then, rather than age, is the physiologically significant event.

Energy Intake

Although the EARs for intake of thiamin, riboflavin, and niacin are not set based on energy intake (IOM, 1998b), it may be appropriate to evaluate intake of these vitamins as a ratio to energy intake for some populations.

The DRI report on the recommended intakes for the B vitamins (IOM, 1998b) notes that no studies were found that examined the effect of energy intake on the requirements for thiamin, riboflavin, or niacin and thus these EARs and RDAs were not based on energy intake. Despite this lack of experimental data, the known biochemical functions of these nutrients suggest that adjustments for energy intake may be appropriate, particularly for individuals with very high intakes (such as those engaged in physically demanding occupations or who spend much time training for active sports). Adjustments may also be appropriate for healthy people with low intakes due to physical inactivity or small body sizes.

For thiamin, riboflavin, and niacin, an energy-adjusted EAR may be calculated as the ratio of the EAR to the median energy requirement for an individual or population. Because DRIs have not been set for energy as of the writing of this report, the requirements for energy recommended in the 10th edition of the RDAs (NRC, 1989) can be used. For example, the thiamin EAR for men 19 through 50 years is 1.0 mg/day and for women is 0.9 mg/day. The recommended median energy intake for men and women 24 through 50 years of age is 2,900 and 2,200 kcal/day, respectively (NRC, 1989). Thus, an energy-adjusted thiamin EAR for adults in this age group would be 0.34 mg/1,000 kcal for men and 0.41 mg/1,000 kcal for women. As was suggested in 1989, for adults with intakes below 2,000 kcal/day, the requirement should not be further reduced (i.e., 0.68 mg/day for men and 0.82 mg/day for women).

An energy-adjusted RDA can be calculated from the energy-adjusted EAR by adding two standard deviations of the requirement. For thiamin, the coefficient of variation of the requirement is 10 percent, so the energy-adjusted RDA would be 20 percent higher than the energy-adjusted EAR, or 0.41 mg/1,000 kcal for men and 0.49 mg/1,000 kcal for women.

MINIMIZING ERRORS IN MEASURING DIETARY INTAKES

Factors influencing food and nutrient intakes are often the same as those influencing requirements, such as life stage, body size, lifestyle, genetic determinants, environment, etc. Food availability and culture also influence intakes but are not related to individual biological requirements. Box 8-1 summarizes points to consider in minimizing error in collecting dietary intake data.

Dietary intakes are determined using a variety of research instruments (e.g., 24-hour recall questionnaires, food records, food-frequency questionnaires, diet histories) that elicit information on types and amounts of food and beverage items consumed. This information is used with values from a nutrient composition database to determine dietary nutrient intake. Contributions of nutrient supplements to dietary intakes are similarly assessed. Following are some techniques for intake measurement that apply to most dietary data collection processes and can help avoid bias and measurement error—and therefore help to ensure the accuracy of individual and group intake measurements. For a more complete review of these issues, see Cameron and Van Staveren (1988), LSRO (1986), NRC (1986), and Thompson and Byers (1994).

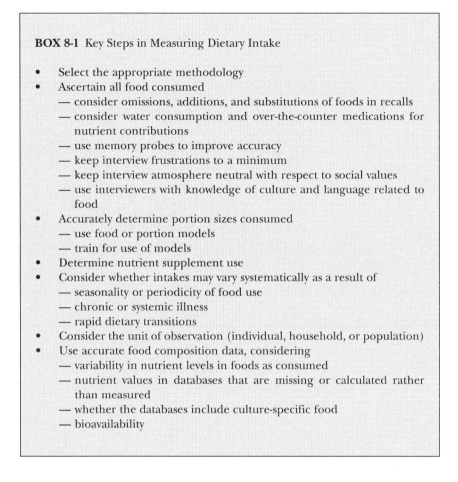

BOX 8-1 Key Steps in Measuring Dietary Intake

- Select the appropriate methodology
- Ascertain all food consumed
  — consider omissions, additions, and substitutions of foods in recalls
  — consider water consumption and over-the-counter medications for nutrient contributions
  — use memory probes to improve accuracy
  — keep interview frustrations to a minimum
  — keep interview atmosphere neutral with respect to social values
  — use interviewers with knowledge of culture and language related to food
- Accurately determine portion sizes consumed
  — use food or portion models
  — train for use of models
- Determine nutrient supplement use
- Consider whether intakes may vary systematically as a result of
  — seasonality or periodicity of food use
  — chronic or systemic illness
  — rapid dietary transitions
- Consider the unit of observation (individual, household, or population)
- Use accurate food composition data, considering
  — variability in nutrient levels in foods as consumed
  — nutrient values in databases that are missing or calculated rather than measured
  — whether the databases include culture-specific food
  — bioavailability

Select the Appropriate Methodology

Dietary intake data are commonly collected using one or more days of recall or records. However, collection of dietary intake data using methods other than a few days of direct reporting of all foods and amounts consumed (e.g., food-frequency questionnaires, diet histories, and household inventories) may appear to be attractive alternatives. Because of the ease of administration and entry of consumption data, semi-quantitative food-frequency questionnaires are widely available and often used in epidemiological studies. These types of questionnaires may be appropriate for ranking intakes in epidemiological studies, but, as noted below, are seldom accurate enough to use to assess the adequacy of dietary intakes of either individuals or groups due to several limiting characteristics of semi-quantitative food frequencies.

First, there is no direct quantitative assessment of individual amounts consumed (Kohlmeier and Bellach, 1995). Either an average portion for all individuals in a group is assumed or the options are limited to a few categories, such as small, medium, and large. Assessment requires a precise quantification of nutrient intakes, and for this, accurate portion sizes are needed. Frequencies of consumption are truncated in a limited number of categories (usually five or seven).

Second, a food-frequency questionnaire does not assess intakes of all available foods. Foods are limited to those that are considered major contributors to the nutrients under study (Block et al., 1986), or to the foods that contributed most to the variance in intake in a specific group at the time the questionnaire was designed (Willett et al., 1987). Food-frequency questionnaires do not attempt to capture all food sources of a nutrient quantitatively.

Third, because of the discrepancy between thousands of foods being offered in a supermarket and a set of questions limited to a few hundred at most, many foods are combined in one question. Food composition data are averaged in some way across these foods, and the individual who consumes only one or another of these or eats these in other proportions will be incorrectly assessed with the nutrient database being used. As a result intakes may be either over- or underestimated. Also often overlooked is that food-frequency questionnaires are only applicable to the population for which they are designed and are based on their consumption patterns at a specific time. Continually changing food consumption patterns and new food offerings require that periodic changes be made in food-frequency questionnaires.

Diet histories, like food frequencies, attempt to capture usual diet but, unlike food frequencies, include quantitative assessment of portions and include the assessment of all foods eaten in a cognitively supportive fashion (meal by meal) (Burke, 1947). Because they are quantitative and do not truncate information on frequency, amount, or the actual food items consumed, diet histories overcome many of the limitations of food-frequency questionnaires for assessment of the total nutrient intakes of individuals (Kohlmeier and Bellach, 1995). Diet histories have also been shown to capture total energy intake more accurately than other methods (Black et al., 1993). However, if conducted by an interviewer, rather than a preset computer program, they may show between-interviewer differences in responses (Kohlmeier et al., 1997).

Household inventories are weak measures of total food intake because of food waste, food consumed by guests or pets, and the large amount of food consumed outside of the home. They also require assumptions about the distribution of food consumption among the people within a household when the household includes more than one person.

Maintaining weighed food records over multiple days can provide a solid basis for nutrient assessment as long as the recording of food intake does not influence usual intake behavior and as long as seasonality in nutrient intake, where it exists, is adequately captured.

In summary, intakes assessed by 24-hour recall, diet records, or quantitative diet histories remain the strongest bases for quantitative assessment of nutrient adequacy using the Dietary Reference Intakes (DRIs). Quantitative assessments require both accurate determination of the quantities of foods consumed by an individual and inclusion of all of the foods that contribute even modestly (more than 5 percent) to the total nutrient intake. Not all dietary intake instruments are designed to meet these requirements. Their use for this purpose is likely to result in inaccurate assessments.

Ascertain All Foods Consumed

Either because of poor memory or a reluctance to report foods felt to be inappropriate, people often omit, add, or substitute foods when recalling or reporting dietary data. On average, total energy intake tends to be underreported by about 20 percent, although the degree of underreporting varies with weight status, body mass index, etc. (Johnson et al., 1998; Lichtman et al., 1992; Mertz et al., 1991). The most common additional food items that were remembered after prompting in the U.S. Department of Agriculture's Continuing Survey of Food Intake by Individuals (1994–1996, Day 1) were beverages, including alcoholic beverages, and snack food, with 5 to 10 percent of nutrient totals being added after prompting (B. Perloff, U.S. Department of Agriculture, unpublished observations, 1998). If foods—and therefore nutrients—are underreported, then the prevalence of inadequate intakes for a population or the probability of inadequacy for an individual may be overestimated. Little is known about the relative sizes of nutrient versus energy under-reporting.

Various techniques may be used to encourage accurate reporting. Because many studies of dietary intake rely on subjects' memory of food, food ingredients, and portion sizes, dietary survey instruments often specify the use of memory probes and cues to improve accuracy (Domel, 1997). Those with poor memory, such as some elderly adults and young children, are not good candidates for dietary intake interviews (Van Staveren et al., 1994; Young, 1981).

Some retrospective diet studies depend on the individual's long-term recall of past food intake and rely on memory that is more generic than that for recent intake. Complete food lists and probes using specific circumstances of life are helpful in these studies (Dwyer and Coleman, 1997; Kuhnlein, 1992; Smith et al., 1991a). The interview atmosphere should be kept neutral so that respondents do not feel they must report (or not report) items because of their social desirability (Hebert et al., 1997).

When dietary intakes are assessed for individuals with strong cultural or ethnic identities, it is useful to employ interviewers from the same background who speak the language of the interviewees and can knowledgeably guide dietary information exchange about the food, its ingredients, and portion sizes. Food composition databases used should contain the appropriate culture-specific food items. Respondents must be literate if written survey instruments are used (Hankin and Wilkens, 1994; Kuhnlein et al., 1996; Teufel, 1997).

Accurately Determine Portion Sizes Consumed

To minimize portion size as a source of error, various kinds of food models, portion-size models, and household measures have been used to assist the respondent (Burk and Pao, 1976; Guthrie, 1984; Haraldsdottir et al., 1994; Thompson et al., 1987; Tsubono et al., 1997). Training the interviewer in use of portion-size models improves accuracy of reporting (Bolland et al., 1990).

Determine Nutrient Supplement Use

Supplement use needs to be determined, and quantified, to obtain accurate estimates of the prevalence of inadequate nutrient intakes for a group. Otherwise, the prevalence of inadequacy will be over-estimated, as will the probability of inadequacy for an individual. However, the proportion of individuals with intakes above the

Tolerable Upper Intake Level (UL) may be underestimated. The extent of under- or overestimation will depend on the dosages and frequency of use, and for groups, on the percentage of the group using supplements. Currently, the only national surveys available which quantify supplement usage along with dietary nutrient intakes are the 1987 National Health Interview Survey and the Third National Health and Nutrition Examination Survey.

Merging two different databases—one dealing with food use and the other dealing with supplement use—to estimate the distribution of usual total intakes is complex because supplements provide relatively high doses of specific nutrients but may be taken intermittently. More accurate methods for measuring nutrient supplement intake are needed.

When assessing adequacy of intake, it may be helpful to average supplement intake over time when the supplement is consumed intermittently (e.g., once per week or month). This will mask or smooth out the high intake associated with the day the supplement was actually consumed. This smoothing effect might be appropriate when assessing for chronic high intakes using the UL. However, if acute effects on health are possible from excessive intake of a nutrient, then a different approach to combining food and supplement intake needs to be proposed. An additional drawback of smoothing supplement intakes is that the day-to-day variability in nutrient intake cannot be estimated. This creates a problem when estimating the usual nutrient intake distribution in a group.

Consider Whether Intakes May Vary Systematically

When dietary intakes of a population or a population subset (e.g., athletes in training) vary systematically, reasons for this variation must be understood and incorporated into data gathering. These techniques also are part of defining what is usual intake (for example, over a calendar year). If systematic variations are not considered, prevalence of inadequate intakes may be under- or overestimated.

Seasonality and Other Issues of Periodicity

Seasonal effects on dietary intakes are reflected in changing patterns of food availability and use. These effects are usually greater for food items than for energy or nutrients (Hartman et al., 1996; Joachim, 1997; Van Staveren et al., 1986). The season of collecting yearly dietary data may bias results because the data will selectively overemphasize items consumed during the season of the interview

(Subar et al., 1994). Seasonally available local cultural food may affect seasonal and yearly average nutrient intakes (Kuhnlein et al., 1996; Receveur et al., 1997). The effects of seasonality on estimated nutrient intakes can be alleviated by a well-designed data collection plan.

Within-person variability also may include other nonrandom components (Tarasuk and Beaton, 1992), some of which may be related to sociocultural factors (e.g., intakes may differ between weekdays and weekend days) (Beaton et al., 1979; Van Staveren et al., 1982) and some of which is physiological (e.g., women's energy intakes vary across the menstrual cycle) (Barr et al., 1995; Tarasuk and Beaton, 1991a).

Illness and Eating Practices

Chronic illness affecting intakes of a part of the population is reflected in group dietary intakes and may bias the prevalence of inadequate intakes in what is assumed to be a normal, healthy population (Kohlmeier et al., 1995; McDowell, 1994; Van Staveren et al., 1994). Parasitism, eating disorders, and dieting—which may be prevalent in segments of a population—may affect food intake. Unlike dieting, illness presents a problem not only with regard to intake data but also in the assumptions underpinning the assessment of adequacy because the DRIs were established for normal, healthy populations.

Rapid Dietary Transition Including Effects of Interventions

Data may be biased by individuals whose dietary intakes are affected by rapidly changing life circumstances (such as migration or refugee status) or by successfully implemented nutrition intervention programs. Thus, it is important to consider how many affected individuals are included in the data sample (Crane and Green, 1980; Immink et al., 1983; Kristal et al., 1990, 1997; Yang and Read, 1996).

Consider the Unit of Observation (Individual, Household, or Population)

Data on nutrient intakes are sometimes collected for households rather than for individuals. When this is the case, the level of aggregation of the dietary data must be matched with an appropriate level of aggregation for the requirements. Appendix E discusses how requirement data may be aggregated at the household level. It is sometimes of interest to compare population-level consumption data (such as food disappearance data for a country) with a requirement estimate. Appropriate ways to make such comparisons are also discussed in Appendix E. However, the methods involve many assumptions, and errors may be large.

Use Accurate Food Composition Data

Deriving nutrient intake data from dietary intake data requires the use of a food composition database. Accuracy of the food composition data and the software to access it are critical for assessments of dietary adequacy. Nutrient databases need to be kept current and contain data on dietary supplements. In the United States and Canada the primary sources of nutrient composition data are the U.S. Department of Agriculture Nutrient Database for Standard Reference, Release 13 and its revisions (USDA, 1999; Watt et al., 1963).

Databases should be evaluated for the number of food items included that are relevant to the population under study (Kuhnlein and Soueida, 1992; Smith et al., 1991b). The currency of data for foods derived from recipes is important; they should reflect changes in fortification levels of primary ingredients. Ideally, the database should not have missing values, and values calculated from similar food items should be identified (Buzzard et al., 1991; Juni, 1996; Nieman et al., 1992).

Other considerations when evaluating databases include whether the values are for food as consumed (rather than as purchased); nutrient analytical methodology used, including extent of sampling required and feasibility of addressing variability in nutrient content; and conventions and modes of data expression (Greenfield and Southgate, 1992; Rand et al., 1991).

When accurate food consumption data are not available, it may be more meaningful to compare food intake to food-based dietary standards (such as the Food Guide Pyramid [USDA, 1992]) than to compare nutrient intake to the DRIs.

Other Factors to Consider

For nutrients with a wide range of biological availability in food, a population's prevalence of inadequate intakes will be inaccurately estimated if the average bioavailability for foods chosen by individuals in the population differs from the bioavailability assumed when setting the Estimated Average Requirement (EAR). The distribution of nutrient intakes also may be inaccurate if bioavailability varies within the population but is not considered when nutrient intake is estimated for each individual. Zinc, niacin, iron, and provitamin A carotenoids are nutrients with well-known issues of bioavailability. Nutrient equivalents are sometimes used (e.g., niacin equivalents for assessing niacin intake and retinol equivalents for assessing intakes of provitamin A carotenoids) (IOM, 1998b, 2000). The use of dietary folate equivalents to reflect the bioavailability of supplemental folate in contrast to folate naturally present in food has been recommended for evaluating dietary data (IOM, 1998b).

ISSUES OF VARIANCE IN DIETARY ASSESSMENT

Selecting a Representative Subsample of a Group

For large groups of people, it is not usually practical to assess the intake of every individual. Thus, a representative subsample is selected and assessed and the findings are extended to the full population. The methods used for ensuring that a sample is truly representative can be complex, but the results of an assessment can be misleading if the individuals who are assessed differ from the rest of the group in either intakes or requirements. Errors can arise if the sample is nonrepresentative. For example, a telephone survey might select more high-income participants by missing families who are too poor to own a telephone. Alternatively, the people who refuse to participate are not a random subsample (e.g., working mothers might be much more likely to refuse than retired people). Therefore, assistance from a statistician or other expert in survey sampling and design should be obtained (Dwyer, 1999; Van Staveren et al., 1994).

Determining Standard Deviations of Prevalence Estimates

Is the estimated prevalence of nutrient inadequacy in a population significantly different from zero?

Answering this question requires estimating the standard deviations associated with the prevalence estimates.

The prevalence estimates obtained from the application of either the probability approach or the Estimated Average Requirement (EAR) cut-point method are exactly that: estimates. As such, there is uncertainty associated with them and this uncertainty can, in principle, be reflected in a standard deviation for the prevalence. Uncertainty in the prevalence estimates can come from three sources: sampling variability, variability associated with the EAR, and variability associated with collection of intake data.

Sampling Variability

Any time a sample of individuals is used to make inferences about a larger group, a statistical error (often called sampling variability) is incurred. In the case of dietary assessment, not only are the intake data obtained for just a sample of individuals in the group, but also the sample of intake days is small for each of those individuals. Therefore, two sources of sampling variability are immediately identifiable—one arising from not observing the entire population and one arising from not observing intake on all days for each individual.

Statistical techniques can be used to estimate the amount of sampling variability associated with prevalence estimates, although the computations are complex. When standard deviations can be calculated, it is appropriate to report not only the prevalence estimate but also its standard deviation. For example, for group X the prevalence of inadequate intake of nutrient Y was a percent ± b percent, where a is the estimated percent prevalence of nutrient inadequacy and b is the standard deviation of the prevalence estimate. When b is small relative to a, the prevalence has been estimated with a good degree of accuracy.

An additional consideration when determining the sampling variability is the effect of the survey design. Dietary intake data are typically collected in complex surveys, and thus the survey design must be taken into account when estimating standard deviations. Additional information on the estimation of standard deviations under complex survey designs, or in particular, about the estimation of standard deviations for prevalence estimates can be found in Nusser et al. (1996) and Wolter (1985).

Variability Associated with the EAR

Variability associated with the EAR may increase the uncertainty around prevalence estimates. Both the probability approach and the cut-point method use the EAR when estimating prevalence of inadequacy. However, the EAR is itself an estimate, and thus has its own uncertainty. Practical statistical approaches have not yet been developed for combining the two uncertainties—those around intake estimates and those around requirement estimates—into a single value that reflects the uncertainty around the prevalence estimate.

Variability Associated with the Collection of Intake Data

Other characteristics of dietary studies complicate the matter even further. Dietary intake data suffer from inaccuracies due to underreporting of food, incorrect specification of portion sizes, incomplete or imprecise food composition tables, etc. These factors may have a compound effect on prevalence estimates. In addition, systematic errors in measurement (such as energy underreporting) may increase the bias of the prevalence estimate. All of these factors have an effect on how precisely (or imprecisely) the prevalence of nutrient adequacy in a group can be estimated, and it is difficult to quantify their effect with confidence.

The software developed at Iowa State University (called SIDE) (Dodd, 1996) to estimate usual intake distributions also produces prevalence estimates using the cut-point method and provides an estimate of the standard deviation associated with the prevalence estimate. *However, it is important to remember that the standard deviations produced by the program are almost certainly an underestimate of the true standard deviations because they do not consider variability associated with the EAR or with the collection of intake data.*

Why should standard deviations be a concern?

Standard deviations of prevalence estimates are needed to determine, for example, whether a prevalence estimate differs from zero or any other target value or to compare two prevalence estimates.

The evaluation of differences in intakes requires the estimation of standard deviations of quantities such as prevalence of nutrient inadequacy or excess (e.g., Application 3 in Chapter 7). As another example, suppose that prevalence of inadequate intake of a nutrient in a group was measured at one point in time as 45 percent. An intervention is applied to the group and then a new estimate of the prevalence of inadequate intake of the nutrient is found to be 38 percent, a decrease of 7 percent. However, to accurately assess the effectiveness of the intervention, the standard deviations around the 45 and 38 percent prevalence estimates are also needed. If the standard deviations are small (e.g., 1 percent), then one could conclude that the intervention was associated with a statistically significant decrease in the prevalence of inadequacy. If the standard deviations are large (e.g., 10 percent), then one could not conclude that the 7 percent decrease was significant or that the intervention worked.

Finally, the part of the intake distribution being assessed affects the error associated with the estimate. Values in the tail of the distribution are harder to estimate (i.e., estimates are less precise) than values in the center of a distribution (such as means or medians). Thus, estimating prevalence of inadequacy of a nutrient is expected to be less precise for nutrients for which prevalence of inadequacy in the group is very low or very high (e.g., 5 or 95 percent) compared with nutrients for which prevalence of inadequacy is towards the center of the distribution (e.g., 30 to 70 percent) for the same sampling design and same estimation method.

SUMMARY

Users of the Dietary Reference Intakes (DRIs) have many opportunities to minimize errors when assessing group and individual intakes. This chapter has focused on ways to increase the accuracy of both the requirement estimates (by considering the specific characteristics of the individual or the population) and the intake estimates (by ensuring that dietary data are complete, portions are correctly specified, and food composition data are accurate) and the importance of an appropriate sampling plan for group intakes.

Although users of the DRIs should strive to minimize errors, perfection usually is not possible or necessary. Comparing high-quality intake data with tailored requirement data to assess intakes is a meaningful undertaking and can, at a minimum, identify nutrients likely to be either under- or overconsumed by the individual or the group of interest.

9

Research Recommended to Improve the Uses of Dietary Reference Intakes

This report has attempted to provide the necessary information to users of the Dietary Reference Intakes (DRIs) for assessing the intakes of groups and individuals. Readers of the report may notice, however, that at various points only very general guidelines are provided. It is clear that much research is still needed in this area. In this last chapter, therefore, areas are listed in which research results are either unavailable or inconclusive. By highlighting these topics, it is hoped that research on these topics will be undertaken. The topics are not necessarily in order of priority; increased knowledge in any of the areas listed below would be of benefit to those who wish to use the DRIs for dietary assessment.

RESEARCH TO IMPROVE ESTIMATES OF NUTRIENT REQUIREMENTS

Even for nutrients for which an Estimated Average Requirement (EAR) is available, requirement data on which the EAR is based are typically very scarce. Estimated EARs and Recommended Dietary Allowances (RDAs) are often based on just a few experiments or studies with very small sample sizes, and therefore considerable uncertainty exists about the true median and standard deviation of the distribution of requirements within a group. Additional research is needed in this area to:

- improve existing estimates of the EAR and RDA;
- provide better information on requirements so it becomes pos-

sible to establish an EAR (and an RDA) for nutrients for which information is currently insufficient; and

• improve estimates of the distribution of requirements so that the appropriate method for assessing the prevalence of inadequacy for groups can be determined (cut-point method vs. probability approach).

For nutrients currently with an Adequate Intake (AI) (for age groups older than infants), research that allows replacement of the AIs with EARs will allow for additional applications. As discussed in earlier chapters, EARs present more possibilities for assessing individual and group prevalence of inadequacy. Whenever the data permit, EARs rather than AIs should be established.

Although there is need to improve the database of controlled experimental studies relevant to the EAR, there is even greater need to broaden the approach to estimating requirements. Congruence of evidence should be expected from different sources—including epidemiological and clinical investigations as well as experimental and factorial approaches—before being confident with an EAR. What is needed now is action in this direction and both financial and peer support for such approaches.

Establishment of Tolerable Upper Intake Levels (ULs) provides an opportunity to evaluate the risk of adverse effects for individuals and populations, and is an extremely important step forward in assessing intakes. Research should be undertaken to allow ULs to be set for all nutrients. In addition, information on the distribution of the UL (i.e., risk curves) would allow greatly expanded applications of the UL, particularly for population groups. More information is needed on ways to identify and conceptualize the risk of exceeding the UL.

Research on the factors that can alter requirements or upper limits is also needed to enable more accurate applications of the Dietary Reference Intakes (DRIs) to specific individuals and populations. Adjustment factors for considerations such as body size, physical activity, and intakes of energy and other nutrients may be appropriate but are often unknown.

RESEARCH TO IMPROVE THE QUALITY OF DIETARY INTAKE DATA

Much has been written about ways to improve the quality of the intake data on which assessments are based; a number of these issues were discussed in Chapter 8. Some of these topics are revisited now and specific areas in which research is still needed are identified.

Perhaps one of the most important advances to improve application of human nutrient requirement estimates has been the further development and refinement of statistical procedures to reduce if not eliminate the distorting effect of random error in dietary data. What has become apparent in dealing with the random error is that the remaining issue of paramount importance in dietary data collection and analysis is the presence and true extent of bias (such as under- or over-reporting of food intake). The same amount of effort that went into determining statistical approaches for estimation and reduction of the effect of random error should be directed toward the estimation and amelioration of bias. This is a relatively unexplored field. Methods for directly estimating bias regarding energy intake have been developed and used to demonstrate that the problem is serious. Efforts have begun in the management of bias during data analysis but these are far from satisfactory at present. The handling of bias is seen as a very high-priority area awaiting new initiatives and innovative approaches.

Another area of need is behavioral research to determine why people under-report food intake. Advances in this area would allow development of improved dietary data collection tools that would not trigger this behavior. Such information would also help in the derivation of statistical tools to correct the bias associated with this phenomenon.

Better ways to quantify the intake of supplements are needed. Methods for collecting accurate supplement intake data have not been widely investigated. For the Third National Health and Nutrition Examination Survey, different instruments were used to collect food intake data and supplement intake data, and the correct methodology for combining these data is uncertain. Furthermore, the intake distribution from supplements usually cannot be adjusted because the current data do not permit the estimation of the day-to-day variability in supplement intake. Despite the difficulties in maintaining a supplement composition database for the rapidly changing market, investigation of better methods of quantifying supplement intakes is a high-priority research area.

Food composition databases need to be updated to include the forms and units that are specified by Dietary Reference Intakes (DRIs). Chemical methodology to facilitate analysis of various forms of certain nutrients (e.g., α- vs. γ-tocopherol) may be required. The DRI recommendations also imply that databases need to separate nutrients inherent in foods from those provided by fortification, particularly when intakes are compared with the Tolerable Upper Intake Level (UL) for nutrients such as niacin. For some nutrients, it may also be necessary to change the units of measurement (e.g., dietary folate equivalents [DFEs], as suggested for folate [IOM, 1998b] and the milligrams of α-tocopherol, suggested for vitamin E in place of α-tocopherol equivalents [IOM, 2000]).

RESEARCH TO IMPROVE STATISTICAL METHODS FOR USING THE DRIs TO ASSESS INTAKES OF INDIVIDUALS

Chapter 3 and Appendix B present an approach to assess the adequacy of an individual's usual intake of nutrients with an Estimated Average Requirement (EAR) or with an Adequate Intake (AI). The following two serious limitations in the application of the method were identified:

• Currently there is not sufficient information to permit calculation of the standard deviation (SD) of daily intake for each individual. It is well known that the SD of daily intake is typically heterogeneous across individuals; however, no research has been conducted to allow the adjustment of a pooled SD estimate to better reflect an individual's daily variability in intakes.
• The approach for testing whether usual intake is greater than requirements (or greater than the AI or less than the Tolerable Upper Intake Level [UL]) makes the critical assumption that daily intakes for an individual are normally distributed. No alternative methodology exists for the many instances in which this assumption is untenable. Research is needed to devise methods for quantitatively assessing individual intakes when the distribution of daily intakes is not symmetrical around the individual's usual intake.

RESEARCH TO IMPROVE STATISTICAL METHODS FOR USING THE DRIs TO ASSESS INTAKES OF GROUPS

The assessment of dietary intake data for groups is challenging because these analyses (presented earlier in this report) do not lend themselves to standard statistical methods. Several methodological issues deserve attention from the scientific community.

Methods for developing standard deviations for prevalence estimates (sometimes referred to as the standard error of the estimate) should be investigated. As discussed in Chapter 8, estimates of the prevalence of inadequacy are not precise because of the uncertainty existing both in requirement estimates and in intake assessments.

When the standard deviation of the prevalence estimate is not known, formal inferences cannot be made about the prevalence of nutrient inadequacy in a group; for example, one cannot determine whether a prevalence estimate differs from zero, or whether prevalence estimates in two groups are different. The statistical approaches included in this report can be used to partially estimate the standard deviation of a prevalence estimate, but these approaches account only for the uncertainty in the estimates of usual intakes in the group.

Uncertainty also exists in requirement estimates. Although the Estimated Average Requirement (EAR) is a fixed and known quantity, based on data reported in the scientific literature, it is also an estimate of an unobservable median requirement for a group. Statistical methods for estimating the standard deviation of the EAR and the standard deviation of the usual intake distribution are, in principle, available. More difficult from a statistical point of view is combining the two sources of uncertainty into an estimate of the standard deviation for the prevalence of nutrient inadequacy.

Research is needed on ways to better match the biomarkers used to set requirements with the effect of dietary intake on those same biomarkers. Research is also needed on the appropriate biochemical data to collect so that these data can be combined with dietary intake data in assessment. Biomarker and other biochemical data are usually too expensive, time-consuming, or both, to collect on large numbers of individuals. However, when this information is available, it can be used in combination with intake data to give a more accurate estimate of the probability of inadequacy. Because biomarker and intake data are very different proxies for the same unobservable variable (nutrient status), combining the information they provide into an estimate of nutritional status for each individual in a group is a challenging statistical task.

Additional research is also needed for applications that assess the nutrient intakes of different subgroups of the population. In particular, evaluations of nutrition assistance programs typically compare nutrient intakes for program participants and a similar group of nonparticipants. A difficult and not fully explored research question is how to estimate differences in the prevalence of inadequacy between subgroups, after controlling for other factors that also affect nutrient intake. Chapter 7 describes a possible approach to addressing this question based on multiple regression analysis, but research is needed to apply this approach to existing survey data sets such as the Continuing Survey of Food Intakes by Individuals and the National Health and Nutrition Examination Surveys.

Ways to assess the performance of methods used to estimate the prevalence of inadequacy should be investigated. Both the probability approach and the cut-point method assume that intakes and requirements are not correlated or exhibit only low correlation. In addition, the cut-point method requires that the distribution of requirements in the population is approximately symmetrical and that the variability of intakes is larger than the variability of requirements. The results presented in Appendix D (that assess the performance of the EAR cut-point method for estimating the prevalence of inadequate intakes) are from simulation studies that should be considered preliminary. A detailed investigation of the effect of violating these assumptions was beyond the scope of this report, but is a high research priority. This investigation would best be done using well-designed, well-planned, and well-implemented simulation studies. This type of study would permit recommendations to be made regarding the best approach for assessing each nutrient and would provide an estimate of the expected bias in prevalence estimates when the conditions for application of the cut-point method are not ideal.

Many of the statistical approaches suggested in this report for adjusting intake distributions and estimating the prevalence of inadequacy for groups can only be implemented with the aid of computer software. Although initial efforts have been made to develop these types of programs, a wider variety of software that can assist users of the Dietary Reference Intakes (DRIs) in correctly applying the methods recommended in this report is needed. There is also a need to upgrade the software used in dietary assessment to incorporate the appropriate statistical methodology described in this report.

10
References

Aickin M, Ritenbaugh C. 1991. Estimation of the true distribution of vitamin A intake by the unmixing algorithm. *Communications Stat Simulations* 20:255–280.

Aksnes L, Aarskog D. 1982. Plasma concentrations of vitamin D metabolites in puberty: Effect of sexual maturation and implications for growth. *J Clin Endocrinol Metab* 55:94–101.

Aloia JF, Vaswani A, Yeh JK, Ross PL, Flaster E, Dilmanian FA. 1994. Calcium supplementation with and without hormone replacement therapy to prevent postmenopausal bone loss. *Ann Intern Med* 120:97–103.

AR (Army Regulation) 40-25. 1985. *See* U.S. Departments of the Army, the Navy, and the Air Force, 1985.

Baran D, Sorensen A, Grimes J, Lew R, Karellas A, Johnson B, Roche J. 1990. Dietary modification with dairy products for preventing vertebral bone loss in premenopausal women: A three-year prospective study. *J Clin Endocrinol Metab* 70:264–270.

Barr SI, Janelle KC, Prior JC. 1995. Energy intakes are higher during the luteal phase of ovulatory menstrual cycles. *Am J Clin Nutr* 61:39–43.

Basiotis PP, Welsh SO, Cronin FJ, Kelsay JL, Mertz W. 1987. Number of days of food intake records required to estimate individual and group nutrient intakes with defined confidence. *J Nutr* 117:1638–1641.

Beaton GH. 1991. Interpretation of results from dietary studies. In: Kohlmeier L, ed. *The Diet History Method: Proceedings of the 2nd Berlin Meeting on Nutritional Epidemiology.* London: Smith-Gordon/Nishimura. Pp. 15–38.

Beaton GH. 1994. Criteria of an adequate diet. In: Shils ME, Olson JA, Shike M, eds. *Modern Nutrition in Health and Disease,* 8th edition. Philadelphia: Lea & Febiger. Pp. 1491–1505.

Beaton GH. 1999. Recommended dietary intakes: Individuals and populations. In: Shils ME, Olson JA, Shike M, Ross AC, eds. *Modern Nutrition in Health and Disease,* 9th edition. Baltimore: Williams & Wilkins. Pp. 1705–1725.

Beaton GH, Chery A. 1988. Protein requirements of infants: A reexamination of concepts and approaches. *Am J Clin Nutr* 48:1403–1412.

Beaton GH, Milner J, Corey P, McGuire V, Cousins M, Stewart E, deRamos M, Hewitt D, Grambsch PV, Kassim N, Little JA. 1979. Sources of variance in 24-hour dietary recall data: Implications for nutrition study design and interpretation. *Am J Clin Nutr* 32:2546–2559.

Beaton GH, Milner J, McGuire V, Feather TE, Little JA. 1983. Source of variance in 24-hour dietary recall data: Implications for nutrition study design and interpretation. Carbohydrate sources, vitamins, and minerals. *Am J Clin Nutr* 37:986–995.

Black AE, Prentice AM, Goldberg GR, Jebb SA, Bingham SA, Livingstone MB, Coward WA. 1993. Measurements of total energy expenditure provide insights into the validity of dietary measurements of energy intake. *J Am Diet Assoc* 93:572–579.

Block G, Hartman AM, Dresser CM, Carroll MD, Gannon J, Gardner L. 1986. A data-based approach to diet questionnaire design and testing. *Am J Epidemiol* 124:453–469.

Bolland JE, Ward JY, Bolland TW. 1990. Improved accuracy of estimating food quantities up to 4 weeks after training. *J Am Diet Assoc* 90:1402–1404, 1407.

Bull NL, Buss DH. 1982. Biotin, panthothenic acid and vitamin E in the British household food supply. *Hum Nutr Appl Nutr* 36:190–196.

Burk MC, Pao EM. 1976. Methodology for large-scale surveys of household and individual diets. *Home Econ Res Rep* No. 40. Washington, DC: Agricultural Research Service/U.S. Department of Agriculture.

Burke BS. 1947. The dietary history as a tool in research. *J Am Diet Assoc* 23:1041–1046.

Buzzard IM, Price KS, Warren RA. 1991. Considerations for selecting nutrient-calculation software: Evaluation of the nutrient database. *Am J Clin Nutr* 54:7–9.

Cameron ME, Van Staveren W. 1988. *Manual on Methodology for Food Consumption Studies.* New York, NY: Oxford University Press.

Canadian Council on Nutrition. 1938. *Canadian Dietary Standards.* Ottawa: Department of Pensions and National Health.

Carriquiry AL. 1999. Assessing the prevalence of nutrient inadequacy. *Public Health Nutr* 2:23–33.

Carriquiry AL, Dodd KW, Nusser SM. 1997. Estimating Adjusted Intake and Biochemical Measurement Distributions for NHANES III. Final report prepared for the National Center for Health Statistics.

Chan GM, Hoffman K, McMurry M. 1995. Effects of dairy products on bone and body composition in pubertal girls. *J Pediatr* 126:551–556.

Chen C. 1999. Spline Estimators of the Distribution Function of a Variable Measured with Error. Unpublished PhD dissertation. Department of Statistics, Iowa State University, Ames.

Chevalley T, Rizzoli R, Nydegger V, Slosman D, Rapin CH, Michel JP, Vasey H, Bonjour JP. 1994. Effects of calcium supplements on femoral bone mineral density and vertebral fracture rate in vitamin-D-replete elderly patients. *Osteoporos Int* 4:245–252.

COMA (Committee on Medical Aspects of Food Policy). 1991. *Dietary Reference Values for Food Energy and Nutrients for the United Kingdom. Report on Health and Social Subjects,* No. 41. London: Her Majesty's Stationery Office.

Crane NT, Green NR. 1980. Food habits and food preferences of Vietnamese refugees living in northern Florida. *J Am Diet Assoc* 76:591–593.

Dabeka RW, McKenzie AD, Conacher HBS, Kirkpatrick DC. 1982. Determination of fluoride in Canadian infant foods and calculation of fluoride intakes by infants. *Can J Public Health* 73:188–191.

Dabeka RW, McKenzie AD, Lecroix GM. 1987. Dietary intakes of lead, cadmium, arsenic and fluoride by Canadian adults: A 24-hour duplicate diet study. *Food Addit Contam* 4:89–101.

Dawson-Hughes B, Dallal GE, Krall EA, Sadowski L, Sahyoun N, Tannenbaum S. 1990. A controlled trial of the effect of calcium supplementation on bone density in postmenopausal women. *N Engl J Med* 323:878–883.

Dawson-Hughes B, Dallal GE, Krall EA, Harris S, Sokoll LJ, Falconer G. 1991. Effect of vitamin D supplementation on wintertime and overall bone loss in healthy postmenopausal women. *Ann Intern Med* 115:505–512.

Dawson-Hughes B, Harris SS, Krall EA, Dallal GE, Falconer G, Green CL. 1995. Rates of bone loss in postmenopausal women randomly assigned to one of two dosages of vitamin D. *Am J Clin Nutr* 61:1140–1145.

Demirjian A. 1980. *Anthropometry Report. Height, Weight, and Body Dimensions: A Report from Nutrition Canada.* Ottawa: Minister of National Health and Welfare, Health and Promotion Directorate, Health Services and Promotion Branch.

Dewey KG, Beaton GH, Fjeld C, Lonnerdal B, Reeds P. 1996. Protein requirements of infants and children. *Eur J Clin Nutr* 50:S119–S150.

Dodd KW. 1996. *A Technical Guide to C-SIDE: Software for Intake Distribution Estimation Version 1.0.* Technical Report 96-TR 32. Ames, IA: Center for Agricultural and Rural Development, Iowa State University.

Domel SB. 1997. Self-reports of diet: How children remember what they have eaten. *Am J Clin Nutr* 65:1148S–1152S.

Dwyer J. 1999. Dietary assessment. In: Shils ME, Olson JA, Shike M, Ross AC, eds. *Modern Nutrition in Health and Disease*, 9th edition. Baltimore: Williams & Wilkins. Pp. 937–959.

Dwyer JT, Coleman KA. 1997. Insights into dietary recall from a longitudinal study: Accuracy over four decades. *Am J Clin Nutr* 65:1153S–1158S.

Eckert RS, Carroll RJ, Wang N. 1997. Transformations to additivity in measurement error models. *Biometrics* 53:262–272.

Eissenstat BR, Wyse BW, Hansen RG. 1986. Pantothenic acid status of adolescents. *Am J Clin Nutr* 44:931–937.

Elders PJ, Netelenbos JC, Lips P, van Ginkel FC, Khoe E, Leeuwenkamp OR, Hackeng WH, van der Stelt PF. 1991. Calcium supplementation reduces vertebral bone loss in perimenopausal women: A controlled trial in 248 women between 46 and 55 years of age. *J Clin Endocrinol Metab* 73:533–540.

Elders PJ, Lips P, Netelenbos JC, van Ginkel FC, Khoe E, van der Vijgh WJ, van der Stelt PF. 1994. Long-term effect of calcium supplementation on bone loss in perimenopausal women. *J Bone Miner Res* 9:963–970.

FAO (Food and Agriculture Organization). 1998. *FAO Food Balance Sheets 1994–1996 Average.* Rome: FAO.

FAO/WHO (Food and Agriculture Organization/World Health Organization). 1970. *Requirements of Ascorbic Acid, Vitamin D, Vitamin B$_{12}$, Folate, and Iron.* Report of a Joint FAO/WHO Expert Group. WHO Technical Report Series No. 452. FAO Nutrition Meetings Report Series No. 47. Geneva: WHO.

FAO/WHO (Food and Agriculture Organization/World Health Organization). 1988. *Requirements of Vitamin A, Iron, Folate, and Vitamin B$_{12}$.* Report of a Joint FAO/WHO Expert Consultation. FAO Food and Nutrition Series No. 23. Rome: FAO.

FAO/WHO/UNU (Food and Agriculture Organization/World Health Organization/United Nations University). 1985. *Energy and Protein Requirements.* Report of a Joint FAO/WHO/UNU Expert Consultation. Technical Report Series. No. 724. Geneva: WHO.

Fuller WA. 1987. *Measurement Error Models.* Wiley Series in Probability and Mathematical Statistics. New York: Wiley.

Gibson RS. 1990. *Principles of Nutritional Assessment.* New York: Oxford University Press.

Gibson RS, Gibson IL, Kitching J. 1985. A study of inter- and intrasubject variability in seven-day weighed dietary intakes with particular emphasis on trace elements. *Biol Trace Elem Res* 8:79–91.

Gloth FM III, Gundberg CM, Hollis BW, Haddad JG Jr, Tobin JD. 1995. Vitamin D deficiency in homebound elderly persons. *J Am Med Assoc* 274:1683–1686.

Gordon AR, Devaney BL, Burghardt JA. 1995. Dietary effects of the National School Lunch Program and the School Breakfast Program. *Am J Clin Nutr* 61:221S–231S.

Greenfield H, Southgate DAT. 1992. *Food Composition Data; Production, Management and Use.* London: Elsevier Applied Science.

Greer FR, Searcy JE, Levin RS, Steichen JJ, Steichen-Asche PS, Tsang RC. 1982. Bone mineral content and serum 25-hydroxyvitamin D concentrations in breast-fed infants with and without supplemental vitamin D: One-year follow-up. *J Pediatr* 100:919–922.

Greger JL, Baligar P, Abernathy RP, Bennett OA, Peterson T. 1978. Calcium, magnesium, phosphorus, copper, and manganese balance in adolescent females. *Am J Clin Nutr* 31:117–121.

Guenther PM, Kott PS, Carriquiry AL. 1997. Development of an approach for estimating usual nutrient intake distributions at the population level. *J Nutr* 127:1106–1112.

Gultekin A, Ozalp I, Hasanoglu A, Unal A. 1987. Serum-25-hydroxycholecalciferol levels in children and adolescents. *Turk J Pediatr* 29:155–162.

Guthrie HA. 1984. Selection and quantification of typical food portions by young adults. *J Am Diet Assoc* 84:1440–1444.

Hallberg L, Hogdahl AM, Nilsson L, Rybo G. 1966. Menstrual blood loss—A population study. Variation at different ages and attempts to define normality. *Acta Obstet Gynecol Scand* 45:320–351.

Hankin JH, Wilkens LR. 1994. Development and validation of dietary assessment methods for culturally diverse populations. *Am J Clin Nutr* 59:198S–200S.

Haraldsdottir J, Tjonneland A, Overvad K. 1994. Validity of individual portion size estimates in a food frequency questionnaire. *Int J Epidemiol* 23:787–796.

Hartman AM, Block G, Chan W, Williams J, McAdams M, Banks WL Jr, Robbins A. 1996. Reproducibility of a self-administered diet history questionnaire administered three times over three different seasons. *Nutr Cancer* 25:305–315.

Hasling C, Charles P, Jensen FT, Mosekilde L. 1990. Calcium metabolism in postmenopausal osteoporosis: The influence of dietary calcium and net absorbed calcium. *J Bone Miner Res* 5:939–946.

Health and Welfare Canada. 1990. *Nutrition Recommendations.* The Report of the Scientific Review Committee. Ottawa: Canadian Government Publishing Centre.

Heaney RP, Recker RR. 1982. Effects of nitrogen, phosphorus, and caffeine on calcium balance in women. *J Lab Clin Med* 99:46–55.

Heaney RP, Recker RR, Saville PD. 1977. Calcium balance and calcium requirements in middle-aged women. *Am J Clin Nutr* 30:1603–1611.

Heaney RP, Recker RR, Saville PD. 1978. Menopausal changes in calcium balance performance. *J Lab Clin Med* 92:953–963.

Hebert JR, Ma Y, Clemow L, Ockene IS, Saperia G, Stanek EJ, Merriam PA, Ockene JK. 1997. Gender differences in social desirability and social approval bias in dietary self-report. *Am J Epidemiol* 146:1046–1055.

Hirano M, Honma K, Daimatsu T, Hayakawa K, Oizumi J, Zaima K, Kanke Y. 1992. Longitudinal variations of biotin content in human milk. *Int J Vitam Nutr Res* 62:281–282.

Immink MDC, Sanjur D, Burgos M. 1983. Nutritional consequences of U.S. migration patterns among Puerto Rican women. *Ecol Food Nutr* 13:139–147.

IOM (Institute of Medicine). 1994. *How Should the Recommended Dietary Allowances Be Revised?* Food and Nutrition Board. Washington, DC: National Academy Press.

IOM (Institute of Medicine). 1997. *Dietary Reference Intakes for Calcium, Phosphorus, Magnesium, Vitamin D, and Fluoride.* Washington, DC: National Academy Press.

IOM (Institute of Medicine). 1998a. *Dietary Reference Intakes: A Risk Assessment Model for Establishing Upper Intake Levels for Nutrients.* Washington, DC: National Academy Press.

IOM (Institute of Medicine). 1998b. *Dietary Reference Intakes for Thiamin, Riboflavin, Niacin, Vitamin B_6, Folate, Vitamin B_{12}, Pantothenic Acid, Biotin, and Choline.* Washington, DC: National Academy Press.

IOM (Institute of Medicine). 2000. *Dietary Reference Intakes for Vitamin C, Vitamin E, Selenium, and Carotenoids.* Washington, DC: National Academy Press.

Jackman LA, Millane SS, Martin BR, Wood OB, McCabe GP, Peacock M, Weaver CM. 1997. Calcium retention in relation to calcium intake and postmenarcheal age in adolescent females. *Am J Clin Nutr* 66:327–333.

James WPT, Schofield EC. 1990. *Human Energy Requirements: A Manual for Planners and Nutritionists.* Oxford: Oxford University Press.

Joachim G. 1997. The influence of time on dietary data: Differences in reported summer and winter food consumption. *Nutr Health* 12:33–43.

Johnson RK, Soultanakis RP, Matthews DE. 1998. Literacy and body fatness are associated with underreporting of energy intake in U.S. low-income women using the multiple-pass 24-hour recall: A doubly labeled water study. *J Am Diet Assoc* 98:1136–1140.

Johnston CC, Miller JZ, Slemenda CW, Reister TK, Hui S, Christian JC, Peacock M. 1992. Calcium supplementation and increases in bone mineral density in children. *N Engl J Med* 327:82–87.

Juni RP. 1996. How should nutrient databases be evaluated? *J Am Diet Assoc* 96:120, 122.

Kathman JV, Kies C. 1984. Pantothenic acid status of free living adolescent and young adults. *Nutr Res* 4:245–250.

Kinyamu HK, Gallagher JC, Balhorn KE, Petranick KM, Rafferty KA. 1997. Serum vitamin D metabolites and calcium absorption in normal young and elderly free-living women and in women living in nursing homes. *Am J Clin Nutr* 65:790–797.

Kohlmeier L, Bellach B. 1995. Exposure assessment error and its handling in nutritional epidemiology. *Annu Rev Public Health* 16:43–59.

Kohlmeier L, Simonsen N, Mottus K. 1995. Dietary modifiers of carcinogenesis. *Environ Health Perspect* 103:177–184.

Kohlmeier L, Mendez M, McDuffie J, Miller M. 1997. Computer-assisted self-interviewing: A multimedia approach to dietary assessment. *Am J Clin Nutr* 65:1275S–1281S.

Krall EA, Sahyoun N, Tannenbaum S, Dallal GE, Dawson-Hughes B. 1989. Effect of vitamin D intake on seasonal variations in parathyroid hormone secretion in postmenopausal women. *N Engl J Med* 321:1777–1783.

Kramer L, Osis D, Wiatrowski E, Spenser H. 1974. Dietary fluoride in different areas in the United States. *Am J Clin Nutr* 27:590–594.

Kristal AR, Abrams BF, Thornquist MD, Disogra L, Croyle RT, Shattuck AL, Henry HJ. 1990. Development and validation of a food use checklist for evaluation of community nutrition interventions. *Am J Public Health* 80:1318–1322.

Kristal AR, Feng Z, Coates RJ, Oberman A, George V. 1997. Associations of race/ethnicity, education, and dietary intervention with the validity and reliability of a food frequency questionnaire: The Women's Health Trial Feasibility Study in Minority Populations. *Am J Epidemiol* 146:856–869.

Kuhnlein HV. 1992. Change in the use of traditional foods by the Nuxalk native people of British Columbia. *Ecol Food Nutr* 27:259–282.

Kuhnlein HV, Soueida R. 1992. Use and nutrient composition of traditional Baffin Inuit foods. *J Food Comp Anal* 5:112–126.

Kuhnlein HV, Soueida R, Receveur O. 1996. Dietary nutrient profiles of Canadian Baffin Island Inuit differ by food source, season, and age. *J Am Diet Assoc* 96:155–162.

Leung SSF, Lui S, Swaminathan R. 1989. Vitamin D status of Hong Kong Chinese infants. *Acta Paediatr Scand* 78:303–306.

Lichtman SW, Pisarska K, Berman ER, Pestone M, Dowling H, Offenbacher E, Weisel H, Heshka S, Matthews DE, Heymsfield SB. 1992. Discrepancy between self-reported and actual caloric intake and exercise in obese subjects. *N Engl J Med* 327:1893–1898.

Liu K. 1988. Consideration of and compensation for intra-individual variability in nutrient intakes. In: Kohlmeier L, Helsing E, eds. *Epidemiology Nutrition and Health: Proceedings of the First Berlin Meeting on Nutritional Epidemiology.* London: Smith-Gordon/Nishimura. Pp. 87–106.

Liu K, Stamler J, Dyer A, McKeever J, McKeever P. 1978. Statistical methods to assess and minimize the role of intra-individual variability in obscuring the relationship between dietary lipids and serum cholesterol. *J Chronic Dis* 31:399–418.

Lloyd T, Andon MB, Rollings N, Martel JK, Landis R, Demers LM, Eggli DF, Kieselhorst K, Kulin HE. 1993. Calcium supplementation and bone mineral density in adolescent girls. *J Am Med Assoc* 270:841–844.

Looker AC, Sempos CT, Liu K, Johnson CL, Gunter EW. 1990. Within-person variance in biochemical indicators of iron status: Effects on prevalence estimates. *Am J Clin Nutr* 52:541–547.

LSRO (Life Sciences Research Office). 1986. *Guidelines for Use of Dietary Intake Data.* Bethesda, MD: LSRO/FASEB.

Markestad T, Elzouki AY. 1991. Vitamin D-deficiency rickets in northern Europe and Libya. In: Glorieux FH, ed. *Rickets: Nestle Nutrition Workshop Series,* Vol 21. New York, NY: Raven Press.

Marshall DH, Nordin BEC, Speed R. 1976. Calcium, phosphorus and magnesium requirement. *Proc Nutr Soc* 35:163–173.

Martin AD, Bailey DA, McKay HA. 1997. Bone mineral and calcium accretion during puberty. *Am J Clin Nutr* 66:611–615.

Matkovic V. 1991. Calcium metabolism and calcium requirements during skeletal modeling and consolidation of bone mass. *Am J Clin Nutr* 54:245S–260S.

Matkovic V, Heaney RP. 1992. Calcium balance during human growth: Evidence for threshold behavior. *Am J Clin Nutr* 55:992–996.

Matkovic V, Fontana D, Tominac C, Goel P, Chesnut CH III. 1990. Factors that influence peak bone mass formation: A study of calcium balance and the inheritance of bone mass in adolescent females. *Am J Clin Nutr* 52:878–888.

McClure FJ. 1943. Ingestion of fluoride and dental caries. Quantitative relations based on food and water requirements of children one to twelve years old. *Am J Dis Child* 66:362–369.

McDowell MA. 1994. The NHANES III Supplemental Nutrition Survey of older Americans. *Am J Clin Nutr* 59:224S–226S.

Mertz W, Kelsay JL. 1984. Rationale and design of the Beltsville one-year dietary intake study. *Am J Clin Nutr* 40:1323–1326.

Mertz W, Tsui JC, Judd JT, Reiser S, Hallfrisch J, Morris ER, Steele PD, Lashley E. 1991. What are people really eating? The relation between energy intake derived from estimated diet records and intake determined to maintain body weight. *Am J Clin Nutr* 54:291–295.

Nieman DC, Butterworth DE, Nieman CN, Lee KE, Lee RD. 1992. Comparison of six microcomputer dietary analysis systems with the USDA Nutrient Data Base for Standard Reference. *J Am Diet Assoc* 92:48–56.

NRC (National Research Council). 1941. *Recommended Dietary Allowances: Protein, Calcium, Iron, Vitamin A, Vitamin B (Thiamin), Vitamin C (Ascorbic Acid), Riboflavin, Nicotinic Acid, Vitamin D.* Washington, DC: National Research Council.

NRC (National Research Council). 1968. *Recommended Dietary Allowances,* 7th Ed. Washington, DC: National Academy of Sciences.

NRC (National Research Council). 1980. *Recommended Dietary Allowances,* 9th Ed. Washington, DC: National Academy Press.

NRC (National Research Council). 1986. *Nutrient Adequacy. Assessment Using Food Consumption Surveys.* Washington, DC: National Academy Press.

NRC (National Research Council). 1989. *Recommended Dietary Allowances,* 10th Ed. Washington, DC: National Academy Press.

Nusser SM, Carriquiry AL, Dodd KW, Fuller WA. 1996. A semiparametric transformation approach to estimating usual daily intake distributions. *J Am Stat Assoc* 91:1440–1449.

O'Dowd KJ, Clemens TL, Kelsey JL, Lindsay R. 1993. Exogenous calciferol (vitamin D) and vitamin D endocrine status among elderly nursing home residents in the New York City area. *J Am Geriatr Soc* 41:414–421.

Ohlson MA, Brewer WD, Jackson L, Swanson PP, Roberts PH, Mangel M, Leverton RM, Chaloupka M, Gram MR, Reynolds MS, Lutz R. 1952. Intakes and retentions of nitrogen, calcium and phosphorus by 136 women between 30 and 85 years of age. *Fed Proc* 11:775–783.

Oliveira V, Gunderson C. 2000. *WIC and the Nutrient Intake of Children.* Food Assistance and Nutrition Research Report No. 5. Beltsville, MD: U.S. Department of Agriculture, Economic Research Service, Food and Rural Economics Division.

Ophaug RH, Singer L, Harland BF. 1980a. Estimated fluoride intake of 6-month-old infants in four dietary regions of the United States. *Am J Clin Nutr* 33:324–327.

Ophaug RH, Singer L, Harland BF. 1980b. Estimated fluoride intake of average two-year-old children in four dietary regions of the United States. *J Dent Res* 59:777–781.

Ophaug RH, Singer L, Harland BF. 1985. Dietary fluoride intake of 6-month and 2-year-old children in four dietary regions of the United States. *Am J Clin Nutr* 42:701–707.

Orwoll ES, Oviatt SK, McClung MR, Deftos LJ, Sexton G. 1990. The rate of bone mineral loss in normal men and the effects of calcium and cholecalciferol supplementation. *Ann Intern Med* 112:29–34.

Osis D, Kramer L, Wiatrowski E, Spencer H. 1974. Dietary fluoride intake in man. *J Nutr* 104:1313–1318.

Prince R, Smith M, Dick IM, Price RI, Webb PG, Henderson NK, Harris MM. 1991. Prevention of postmenopausal osteoporosis. A comparative study of exercise, calcium supplementation, and hormone-replacement therapy. *N Engl J Med* 325:1189–1195.

Prince R, Devine A, Dick I, Criddle A, Kerr D, Kent N, Price R, Randell A. 1995. The effects of calcium supplementation (milk powder or tablets) and exercise on bone density in postmenopausal women. *J Bone Miner Res* 10:1068–1075.

Rand WM, Pennington JAT, Murphy SP, Klensin JC. 1991. *Compiling Data for Food Composition Data Bases*. Tokyo: United Nations University Press.

Receveur O, Boulay M, Kuhnlein HV. 1997. Decreasing traditional food use affects diet quality for adult Dene/Metis in 16 communities of the Canadian Northwest Territories. *J Nutr* 127:2179–2186.

Recker RR, Hinders S, Davies KM, Heaney RP, Stegman MR, Lappe JM, Kimmel DB. 1996. Correcting calcium nutritional deficiency prevents spine fractures in elderly women. *J Bone Miner Res* 11:1961–1966.

Reid IR, Ames RW, Evans MC, Gamble GD, Sharpe SJ. 1995. Long-term effects of calcium supplementation on bone loss and fractures in postmenopausal women: A randomized controlled trial. *Am J Med* 98:331–335.

Riis B, Thomsen K, Christiansen C. 1987. Does calcium supplementation prevent postmenopausal bone loss? *N Engl J Med* 316:173–177.

Rose D, Habicht JP, Devaney B. 1998. Household participation in the Food Stamp and WIC programs increases the nutrient intakes of preschool children. *J Nutr* 128:548–555.

Salmenpera L, Perheentupa J, Pispa JP, Siimes MA. 1985. Biotin concentrations in maternal plasma and milk during prolonged lactation. *Int J Vitam Nutr Res* 55:281–285.

Selby PL. 1994. Calcium requirement—A reappraisal of the methods used in its determination and their application to patients with osteoporosis. *Am J Clin Nutr* 60:944–948.

Sempos CT, Johnson NE, Smith EL, Gilligan C. 1985. Effects of intraindividual and interindividual variation in repeated dietary records. *Am J Epidemiol* 121:120–130.

Sims LS. 1996. Uses of the Recommended Dietary Allowances: A commentary. *J Am Diet Assoc* 96:659–662.

Singer L, Ophaug R. 1979. Total fluoride intakes of infants. *Pediatrics* 63:460–466.

Singer L, Ophaug RH, Harland BF. 1980. Fluoride intakes of young male adults in the United States. *Am J Clin Nutr* 33:328–332.

Singer L, Ophaug RH, Harland BF. 1985. Dietary fluoride intake of 15–19-year-old male adults residing in the United States. *J Dent Res* 64:1302–1305.

Smith AF, Jobe JB, Mingay DJ. 1991a. Retrieval from memory of dietary information. *Appl Cognitive Psychol* 5:269–296.

Smith CJ, Schakel SF, Nelson RG. 1991b. Selected traditional and contemporary foods currently used by the Pima Indians. *J Am Diet Assoc* 91:338–341.

Snedecor GW, Cochran WG. 1980. *Statistical Methods*, 7th edition. Ames, Iowa: Iowa State University Press.

Specker BL, Ho ML, Oestreich A, Yin TA, Shui QM, Chen XC, Tsang RC. 1992. Prospective study of vitamin D supplementation and rickets in China. *J Pediatr* 120:733–739.

Spencer H, Kramer L, Lesniak M, DeBartolo M, Norris C, Osis D. 1984. Calcium requirements in humans. Report of original data and a review. *Clin Orthop Relat Res* 184:270–280.

Spencer H, Osis D, Lender M. 1981. Studies of fluoride metabolism in man. A review and report of original data. *Sci Total Environ* 17:1–12.

Srinivasan V, Christensen N, Wyse BW, Hansen RG. 1981. Pantothenic acid nutritional status in the elderly—Institutionalized and noninstitutionalized. *Am J Clin Nutr* 34:1736–1742.

Stefanski LA, Bay JM. 1996. Simulation extrapolation deconvolution of finite population cumulative distribution function estimators. *Biometrika* 83:407–417.

Subar AF, Frey CM, Harlan LC, Kahle L. 1994. Differences in reported food frequency by season of questionnaire administration: The 1987 National Health Interview Survey. *Epidemiology* 5:226–233.

Tarasuk V, Beaton GH. 1991a. Menstrual-cycle patterns in energy and macronutrient intake. *Am J Clin Nutr* 53:442–447.

Tarasuk V, Beaton GH. 1991b. The nature and individuality of within-subject variation in energy intake. *Am J Clin Nutr* 54:464–470.

Tarasuk V, Beaton GH. 1992. Statistical estimation of dietary parameters: Implications of patterns in within-subject variation—A case study of sampling strategies. *Am J Clin Nutr* 55:22–27.

Tarr JB, Tamura T, Stokstad EL. 1981. Availability of vitamin B_6 and pantothenate in an average American diet in man. *Am J Clin Nutr* 34:1328–1337.

Taves DR. 1983. Dietary intake of fluoride ashed (total fluoride) v. unashed (inorganic fluoride) analysis of individual foods. *Br J Nutr* 49:295–301.

Teufel NI. 1997. Development of culturally competent food-frequency questionnaires. *Am J Clin Nutr* 65:1173S–1178S.

Thompson CH, Head MK, Rodman SM. 1987. Factors influencing accuracy in estimating plate waste. *J Am Diet Assoc* 87:1219–1220.

Thompson FE, Byers T. 1994. Dietary assessment resource manual. *J Nutr* 124:2245S–2317S.

Tsubono Y, Kobayashi M, Takahashi T, Iwase Y, Iitoi Y, Akabane M, Tsugane S. 1997. Within- and between-person variations in portion sizes of foods consumed by the Japanese population. *Nutr Cancer* 29:140–145.

USDA (U.S. Department of Agriculture, Human Nutrition Information Service). 1992. The Food Guide Pyramid. Home and Garden Bulletin No. 252, 32 pp.

USDA (U.S. Department of Agriculture, Agricultural Research Service). 1999. USDA Nutrient Database for Standard Reference, Release 13. Nutrient Data Laboratory Home Page. Available from: <http://www.nal.usda.gov/fnic/foodcomp>.

U.S. Departments of the Army, the Navy, and the Air Force. 1985. Army Regulation 40-25/Navy Command Medical Instruction 10110.1/Air Force Regulation 160-95. *Nutritional Allowances, Standards, and Education*. May 15. Washington, D.C.

Van Staveren WA, Hautvast JG, Katan MB, Van Montfort MA, Van Oosten-Van der Goes HG. 1982. Dietary fiber consumption in an adult Dutch population. *J Am Diet Assoc* 80:324–330.

Van Staveren WA, Deurenberg P, Burema J, de Groot LC, Hautvast JG. 1986. Seasonal variation in food intake, pattern of physical activity and change in body weight in a group of young adult Dutch women consuming self-selected diets. *Int J Obes* 10:133–145.

Van Staveren WA, de Groot LC, Blauw YH, van der Wielen RPJ. 1994. Assessing diets of elderly people: Problems and approaches. *Am J Clin Nutr* 59:221S–223S.

Watt BK, Merrill AL, Pecot RK. 1963. *Composition of Foods; Raw, Processed, Prepared.* Agriculture Handbook No. 8. Washington, DC: U.S. Department of Agriculture.

Welsh S, Davis C, Shaw A. 1992. Development of the food guide pyramid. *Nutr Today* 27:12–23.

Willett WC, Reynolds RD, Cottrell-Hoehner S, Sampson L, Browne ML. 1987. Validation of a semi-quantitative food frequency questionnaire: Comparison with a 1-year diet record. *J Am Diet Assoc* 87:43–47.

Wolter KM. 1985. *Introduction to Variance Estimation.* New York: Springer-Verlag.

Yang W, Read M. 1996. Dietary pattern changes of Asian immigrants. *Nutr Res* 16:1277–1293.

Young CM. 1981. Dietary methodology. In: *Assessing Changing Food Consumption Patterns.* Food and Nutrition Board, National Research Council. Washington, DC: National Academy Press. Pp. 89–118.

Zeisel SH, da Costa K-A, Franklin PD, Alexander EA, Lamont JT, Sheard NF, Beiser A. 1991. Choline, an essential nutrient for humans. *FASEB J* 5:2093–2098.

A

Origin and Framework of the Development of Dietary Reference Intakes

This report is one of a series of publications resulting from the comprehensive effort being undertaken by the Food and Nutrition Board's Standing Committee on the Scientific Evaluation of Dietary Reference Intakes and its panels and subcommittees.

ORIGIN

This initiative began in June 1993, when the Food and Nutrition Board (FNB) organized a symposium and public hearing entitled "Should the Recommended Dietary Allowances Be Revised?" Shortly thereafter, to continue its collaboration with the larger nutrition community on the future of the Recommended Dietary Allowances (RDAs), the FNB took two major steps: (1) it prepared, published, and disseminated the concept paper "How Should the Recommended Dietary Allowances Be Revised?" (IOM, 1994), which invited comments regarding the proposed concept, and (2) it held several symposia at nutrition-focused professional meetings to discuss the FNB's tentative plans and to receive responses to this initial concept paper. Many aspects of the conceptual framework of the Dietary Reference Intakes (DRIs) came from the United Kingdom's report *Dietary Reference Values for Food Energy and Nutrients for the United Kingdom* (COMA, 1991).

The five general conclusions presented in the FNB's 1994 concept paper are as follows:

1. Sufficient new information has accumulated to support a

reassessment of the RDAs.

2. Where sufficient data for efficacy and safety exist, reduction in the risk of chronic degenerative disease is a concept that should be included in the formulation of future recommendations.

3. Upper levels of intake should be established where data exist regarding risk of adverse effects.

4. Components of food of possible benefit to health, although not meeting the traditional concept of a nutrient, should be reviewed, and if adequate data exist, reference intakes should be established.

5. Serious consideration must be given to developing a new format for presenting future recommendations.

Subsequent to the symposium and the release of the concept paper, the FNB held workshops at which invited experts discussed many issues related to the development of nutrient-based reference values, and FNB members have continued to provide updates and engage in discussions at professional meetings. In addition, the FNB gave attention to the international uses of the earlier RDAs and the expectation that the scientific review of nutrient requirements should be similar for comparable populations.

Concurrently, Health Canada and Canadian scientists were reviewing the need for revision of the *Recommended Nutrient Intakes* (RNIs) (Health and Welfare Canada, 1990). A consensus was reached following a symposium for Canadian scientists cosponsored by the Canadian National Institute of Nutrition and Health Canada in April 1995. This consensus was that the Canadian government should pursue the extent to which involvement with the developing FNB process would be of benefit to both Canada and the United States in terms of leading toward harmonization.

On the basis of extensive input and deliberations, the FNB initiated action to provide a framework for the development and possible international harmonization of nutrient-based recommendations that would serve, where warranted, for all of North America. To this end, in December 1995, the FNB began a close collaboration with the government of Canada and took action to establish the Standing Committee on the Scientific Evaluation of Dietary Reference Intakes.

THE CHARGE TO THE COMMITTEE

In 1995 the Standing Committee on the Scientific Evaluation of Dietary Reference Intakes (DRI Committee) was appointed to oversee and conduct this project. To accomplish this task, the DRI Committee devised a plan involving the work of expert nutrient group panels and two overarching subcommittees (Figure A-1).

The Subcommittee on Interpretation and Uses of Dietary Reference Intakes (Uses Subcommittee) is composed of experts in nutrition, dietetics, statistics, nutritional epidemiology, public health, economics, and consumer perspectives. The Uses Subcommittee is charged to review the scientific literature regarding the uses of dietary reference standards and their applications and (1) provide guidance for the appropriate application of DRIs for specific purposes and identify inappropriate applications, (2) provide guidance for adjustments to be made for potential errors in dietary intake data and the assumptions regarding intake and requirement distributions, and (3) provide specific guidance for use of DRI values of individual nutrients.

The Uses Subcommittee was charged with examining the appropriate use of each of the DRI values in assessing nutrient intakes of groups and of individuals for this report; a future report will present information on the appropriate use of specific DRI values in the planning of diets for groups and for individuals. Each report will present the statistical underpinnings for the various uses of the DRI values and also will indicate when specific uses are inappropriate. This report reflects the work of the DRI Committee, the Uses Subcommittee, and the Subcommittee on Upper Reference Levels of Nutrients, all under the oversight of the Food and Nutrition Board.

PARAMETERS FOR DIETARY REFERENCE INTAKES

Life Stage Groups

Nutrient intake recommendations are expressed for 16 life stage groups, as listed in Table A-1 and described in more detail in the first Dietary Reference Intake (DRI) nutrient report (IOM, 1997). If data are too sparse to distinguish differences in requirements by life stage and gender group, the analysis may be presented for a larger grouping. Differences will be indicated by gender when warranted by the data.

Reference Heights and Weights

The reference heights and weights selected for adults and children are shown in Table A-2. The values are based on anthropometric data collected from 1988 through 1994 as part of the Third National Health and Nutrition Examination Survey (NHANES III) in the United States.

182

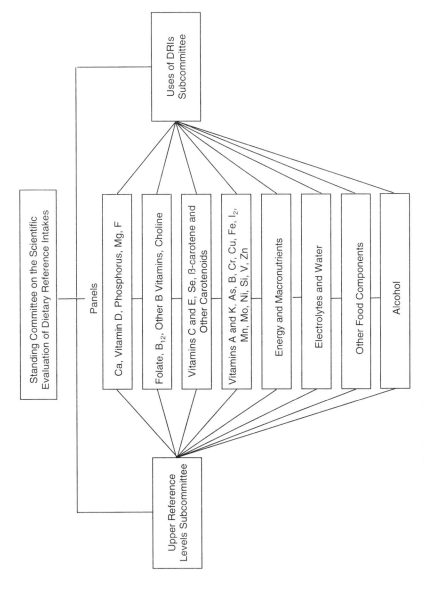

FIGURE A-1 Dietary Reference Intakes project structure.

TABLE A-1 The 16 Life Stage Groups for Which Nutrient Recommendations Are Expressed[a]

Life Stage Groups	
Infants	Females
0–6 mo	9–13 y
7–12 mo	14–18 y
	19–30 y
Children	31–50 y
1–3 y	51–70 y
4–8 y	> 70 y
Males	Pregnancy
9–13 y	≤ 18 y
14–18 y	19–30 y
19–30 y	31–50 y
31–50 y	
51–70 y	Lactation
> 70 y	≤ 18 y
	19–30 y
	31–50 y

[a] Differences will be indicated by gender when warranted by the data.

TABLE A-2 Reference Heights and Weights for Children and Adults in the United States[a]

Gender	Age	Median Body Mass Index	Reference Height cm (in)	Reference Weight[b] kg (lb)
Male, female	2–6 mo	–	64 (25)	7 (16)
	7–11 mo	–	72 (28)	9 (20)
	1–3 y	–	91 (36)	13 (29)
	4–8 y	15.8	118 (46)	22 (48)
Male	9–13 y	18.5	147 (58)	40 (88)
	14–18 y	21.3	174 (68)	64 (142)
	19–30 y	24.4	176 (69)	76 (166)
Female	9–13 y	18.3	148 (58)	40 (88)
	14–18 y	21.3	163 (64)	57 (125)
	19–30 y	22.8	163 (64)	61 (133)

[a] Adapted from the Third National Health and Nutrition Examination Survey, 1988–1994. Body mass index expressed as kg/m^2.

[b] Calculated from body mass index and height for ages 4 through 8 y and older.

The reference weights chosen for this report were based on NHANES III data because these are the most recent data available for either the United States or Canada. The most recent nationally representative data available for Canadians are from the 1970–1972 Nutrition Canada Survey (Demirjian, 1980).

Reference weights are used primarily when setting the Estimated Average Requirement (EAR), Adequate Intake (AI), or Tolerable Upper Intake Level (UL) for children or when relating the nutrient needs of adults to body weight. For the 4- through 8-year-old age group, it can be assumed that a small 4-year-old child will require less than a large 8-year-old. However, the RDA or AI for the 4- through 8-year-old age group should meet the needs of both.

B

Nutrient Assessment of Individuals: Statistical Foundations

Chapter 3 provides an approach that can be used to answer the following question for nutrients with an Estimated Average Requirement (EAR), Can an individual's intake, observed for a small number of days, be used to determine if that individual's *usual* intake of a nutrient is adequate? Similarly, guidance on how to determine, for a given confidence level, whether an individual's usual intake exceeds the Adequate Intake (AI) or the Tolerable Upper Intake Level (UL) is also presented in Chapter 3. The statistical underpinnings and the implementation of the approaches provided are described in this appendix.

To begin, two important terms must be defined:

• The *observed intake* of a nutrient by an individual on a given day is denoted by Y_j, where j denotes the day on which the intake Y was recorded. In this appendix, $j = 1,...,n$, is used to indicate that the number of daily intake observations for an individual can be any number (some arbitrary value n). In practice, n is typically less than seven, and is often no more than two or three. The *observed mean intake* for the individual over the n days is denoted by $\bar{y}$, and is computed as:

$$\bar{y} = (Y_1 + Y_2 + ... + Y_n)/n.$$

• The *usual intake* of a nutrient by an individual is an unobservable *long-run average* intake of the nutrient denoted as y. Conceptually, the usual intake y could be computed as above if the number of

185

intake days (n) available for the individual was very large. In practice an individual's usual intake is seldom known; instead, the individual's observed mean intake $\bar{y}$ is used as an estimate of the individual's usual intake y.

When assessing an individual's dietary intake, *usual* intake and not *observed* intake should be compared with the requirement to determine whether the intake is adequate (or whether it exceeds the UL).

Assessing the adequacy of an individual's intake of a nutrient by using only dietary information is difficult because neither the *usual* intake nor the actual *requirement* of the individual is known. The approach detailed here for assessing the adequacy of an individual's intake requires four types of information: the median requirement of the nutrient for the individual's life stage and gender group (the EAR), the variability in the requirement for the individual's life stage and gender group, the mean observed intake for the individual, and the day-to-day variability in intake of the nutrient for the individual. By combining this information appropriately, a method for estimating the adequacy of an individual's *usual* intake of a nutrient can be derived. A similar approach may be used to compare observed intake to an AI or UL, and will be discussed later in this appendix.

USING THE EAR TO ASSESS ADEQUACY OF AN INDIVIDUAL'S OBSERVED INTAKE

Following are the assumptions for the statistical approach to evaluating the adequacy of an individual's observed intake:

1. The Estimated Average Requirement (EAR) is the best estimate of the individual's *unobservable* true requirement, denoted by ρ. The estimate for the individual's requirement is denoted by r, and r is set to be equal to the EAR of the appropriate life stage and gender group. The standard deviation of requirements in the population, denoted by SD_r is proportional to the uncertainty about how precisely r estimates ρ. If every individual had the exact same requirement for the nutrient, then r (which is set to be equal to the EAR) would be a precise estimate of each individual's requirement. Because individuals vary in their requirement for a nutrient, it is important to consider the extent of the variability in the group; the SD_r is an indicator of how variable requirements are in the group.

2. The mean of n days of intake of the nutrient by the individual, $\bar{y}$, is the best estimate for y, the individual's usual intake. The day-to-day variation in intake for a given individual, also referred to as the within-person standard deviation of daily intakes, SD_{within}, is proportional to the uncertainty about the accuracy of $\bar{y}$ as an estimate of y. The mean ($\bar{y}$) will be a reliable estimate of the usual intake y when the number of intake days n from which the mean was computed is large or when the SD_{within} is low. If an individual eats the same diet day after day, then the day-to-day variability in intakes for that individual would be very low, and one or two days of intake information might be sufficient to precisely estimate that individual's usual intake of the nutrient. Conversely, a large number n of dietary intake observations is needed to estimate the usual intake of a nutrient for an individual whose diet is variable from one day to the next.

It is implicitly assumed that food intake can be measured accurately in terms of quantity of food and food composition. Therefore, results from individual assessments should be interpreted with caution and where possible, should be combined with other interpretive data.

Thus the following statements can be made:

If $y > \rho$, then the individual's usual intake of the nutrient is adequate.

If $y < \rho$, then the individual's usual intake of the nutrient is inadequate.

Because neither y nor ρ is observed, $\bar{y}$ and r must be used instead. Inferences about the adequacy of the individual's diet can be made by looking at the observed difference (D), where

$$D = \bar{y} - r.$$

Intuitively, if D is large and positive, it is likely that the true difference $y - \rho$ is also large and that the individual's diet is adequate. Conversely, if D is a large negative number, then it is likely that ρ is larger than y and that the individual's intake is not adequate. The obvious question to be posed is, How large would D have to be before it can be concluded, with some degree of assurance, that the unobservable usual intake is larger than the unobservable requirement?

To interpret this difference between observed mean intake ($\bar{y}$) and the median requirement (EAR, the best estimate [r] of the unobservable ρ), one needs a measure of the variability of D. The standard deviation of requirements (SD_r) and the standard deviation of intakes (SD_{within} or SD_i) can be used to estimate the SD of D, the difference between observed mean intake and r for the individual, as

$$SD_D = \sqrt{V_r + \left(V_{within} / n \right)}.$$

V_r denotes the *variance* of the distribution of requirements in the group and V_{within} denotes the variance in day-to-day intakes of the nutrient. Both variances are computed as the square of the corresponding standard deviations. As the number (n) of days of intake available on the individual increases, the variance of the observed mean intake should decrease (i.e., the accuracy of the estimate for y increases). This is why V_{within} is divided by n when computing the standard deviation of the difference D.

The SD_D increases as the

- SD_r increases,
- SD_i increases, or
- number of intake days (n) available for the individual decreases.

That is, the more uncertainty that exists about the accuracy of the value D, the larger D will need to be before it can be confidently stated that the individual's *usual* intake is adequate. The following extreme cases illustrate this approach:

1. If the intake of an individual could be observed for a very large (infinite) number of days, then the second term (V_{within}/n) in the expression for SD_D would tend to zero. The uncertainty about the adequacy of the individual's intake would result primarily from not knowing where in the distribution of requirements that individual's unobservable requirement ρ is located. The degree of uncertainty about adequacy would then be proportional to the variability of requirements in the group.

2. If the individual were to consume the same diet day after day, then the second term (V_{within}/n) would again be very small, even with small n, because the variability in intakes from day to day would be very small for that individual. Again, the uncertainty about the

adequacy of the individual's intake would reflect the uncertainty about that individual's requirement for the nutrient.

3. Hypothetically, if an individual's requirement could be observed, then the first term in the expression for SD_D would be zero, and the uncertainty would reflect only the fact that the individual's usual intake for the nutrient cannot be observed.

The three situations above are extreme and typically do not occur. A more common situation is when there is some information about the individual's daily intake (allowing for an estimate of $\bar{y}$) and some idea of the distribution of requirements in the group. For example, the median requirement (EAR) and the coefficient of variation (CV) of requirements might be known, allowing the SD_r to be derived.

Suppose that a level of confidence of at least 85 percent is desired before concluding that an individual's usual intake is adequate. To find out how large the ratio D/SD_D would need to be to reach this conclusion, compare the D/SD_D to the z-values listed in a standard z-table (e.g., a value of 0.85 in the table corresponds to a z-value of 1). Thus, if the ratio D/SD_D is approximately equal to 1, it can be concluded with an 85 percent level of confidence that the individual's usual intake is larger than the requirement. Selected z-values, corresponding to different levels of assurance, are given in Table B-1. The criterion for using the ratio D/SD_D and the qualitative conclusions from the quantitative analysis can be summarized as follows:

- If D/SD_D is greater than 1, then there is reasonable certainty that the individual's usual intake is adequate. In other words, it is reasonably certain that the unobservable true difference between the individual's usual intake and requirement $(y - \rho)$ is positive and thus the individual's usual intake exceeds requirement.
- If D/SD_D is less than –1, then it is reasonably certain that the individual's usual intake is inadequate. In other words, the true difference between the individual's usual intake and requirement $(y - \rho)$ is negative and thus the individual's usual intake is less than the requirement.
- If D/SD_D is anywhere between –1 and 1, it cannot be determined with certainty whether the individual's intake is adequate or inadequate.

The criterion above is derived by using principles from hypothesis testing and construction of confidence intervals under normality

TABLE B-1 Values for the Ratio D/SD_D and Corresponding Probability of Correctly Concluding that Usual Intake Is Adequate or Inadequate

Criterion	Conclusion	Probability of Correct Conclusion
$D/SD_D > 2.00$	Usual intake is adequate	0.98
$D/SD_D > 1.65$	Usual intake is adequate	0.95
$D/SD_D > 1.50$	Usual intake is adequate	0.93
$D/SD_D > 1.00$	Usual intake is adequate	0.85
$D/SD_D > 0.50$	Usual intake is adequate	0.70
$D/SD_D > 0.00$	Usual intake is adequate (inadequate)	0.50
$D/SD_D < -0.50$	Usual intake is inadequate	0.70
$D/SD_D < -1.00$	Usual intake is inadequate	0.85
$D/SD_D < -1.50$	Usual intake is inadequate	0.93
$D/SD_D < -1.65$	Usual intake is inadequate	0.95
$D/SD_D < -2.00$	Usual intake is inadequate	0.98

SOURCE: Adapted from Snedecor and Cochran (1980).

and is only approximate. The assumptions that are implicit in the criterion include:

1. The distribution of daily intakes Y around the mean intake $\bar{y}$ is approximately normal, or at least symmetrical, for the individual. Any nutrient with a skewed distribution of daily intakes would not satisfy this assumption, such as those nutrients in Tables B-2 through B-5 with a CV larger than about 60 to 70 percent.

2. The distribution of requirements in the group is approximately normal.

3. The daily intake Y accurately reflects the individual's true intake of the nutrient for the day.

4. A reliable estimate of the day-to-day variability in intake for the individual is available.

5. Intakes are independent of requirements.

In probabilistic terms, the value of 1 for the ratio D/SD_D corresponds to an approximate 0.15 p-value for the test of the hypothesis that $y > \rho$. That is, when it is concluded that intake is adequate, there is approximately an 85 percent chance of reaching the correct conclusion and approximately a 15 percent chance of making a mistake (erroneously concluding that intake is adequate). Because the criterion is formulated on this probabilistic basis, the level of

TABLE B-2 Estimates of Within-Subject Variation in Intake, Expressed as Standard Deviation $(SD)^a$ and Coefficient of Variation (CV) for Vitamins and Minerals in Adults Aged 19 and Over

Nutrient[b]	Adults Ages 19–50 y				Adults, Ages 51 y and Over			
	Females (n = 2,480)[c]		Males (n = 2,538)		Females (n = 2,162)		Males (n = 2,280)	
	SD	CV (%)	SD	CV (%)	SD	CV (%)	SD	CV (%)
Vitamin A (µg)	1,300	152	1,160	115	1,255	129	1,619	133
Carotene (RE)	799	175	875	177	796	147	919	153
Vitamin E (mg)	5	76	7	176	6	65	9	60
Vitamin C (mg)	73	87	93	92	61	69	72	71
Thiamin (mg)	0.6	47	0.9	46	0.5	41	0.7	40
Riboflavin (mg)	0.6	50	1.0	44	0.6	42	0.8	40
Niacin (mg)	9	47	12	44	7	42	9	39
Vitamin B$_6$ (mg)	0.8	53	1.0	48	0.6	44	0.8	42
Folate (µg)[d]	131	62	180	61	12	52	150	53
Vitamin B$_{12}$ (µg)	12	294	13	212	10	237	14	226
Calcium (mg)	325	51	492	54	256	44	339	44
Phosphorous (mg)	395	39	573	38	313	33	408	32
Magnesium (mg)	86	38	122	38	74	33	94	32
Iron (mg)	7	53	9	51	5	44	7	44
Zinc (mg)	6	61	9	63	5	58	8	66
Copper (mg)	0.6	53	0.7	48	0.5	53	0.7	56
Sodium (mg)	1,839	44	1,819	43	1,016	41	1,323	38
Potassium (mg)	851	38	1,147	36	723	31	922	31

NOTE: When the *CV* is larger than 60 to 70 percent the distribution of daily intakes is nonnormal and the methods presented here are unreliable.

[a] Square root of the residual variance after accounting for subject, and sequence of observation (gender and age controlled by classifications).

[b] Nutrient intakes are for food only, data does not include intake from supplements.

[c] Sample size was inadequate to provide separate estimates for pregnant or lactating women.

[d] Folate reported in µg rather than as the new dietary folate equivalents (DFE).

SOURCE: Data from Continuing Survey of Food Intakes by Individuals 1994–1996.

certainty can be adjusted by either increasing or decreasing the value of the cutoff for D/SD_D (e.g., if 0.5 or –0.5 was used, then the level of certainty would decrease to about 70 percent). Table B-1 indicates the probability, or level of certainty, of correctly concluding that the usual intake is adequate (or inadequate) when D/SD_D ranges from 2.00 to –2.00.

TABLE B-3 Estimates of Within-Subject Variation in Intake, Expressed as Standard Deviation $(SD)^a$ and Coefficient of Variation (CV) for Vitamins and Minerals in Adolescents and Children

Nutrient [b]	Adolescents, Ages 9–18 y				Children, Ages 4–8 y			
	Females ($n = 1,002$)		Males ($n = 998$)		Females ($n = 817$)		Males ($n = 883$)	
	SD	CV (%)	SD	CV (%)	SD	CV (%)	SD	CV (%)
Vitamin A (µg)	852	109	898	91	808	103	723	86
Carotene (RE)	549	180	681	197	452	167	454	166
Vitamin E (mg)	4	67	5	62	3	54	3	57
Vitamin C (mg)	81	90	93	89	61	69	74	76
Thiamin (mg)	0.6	43	0.8	42	0.5	35	0.5	37
Riboflavin (mg)	0.7	42	1.0	41	0.6	35	0.7	35
Niacin (mg)	8	46	11	43	6	36	7	38
Vitamin B$_6$ (µg)	0.7	49	1.0	49	0.6	42	0.7	43
Folate (µg) [c]	128	58	176	60	99	48	117	50
Vitamin B$_{12}$ (µg)	5.5	142	5.0	93	9.6	254	4.7	118
Calcium (mg)	374	48	505	48	313	40	353	41
Phosphorous (mg)	410	38	542	37	321	32	352	32
Magnesium (mg)	86	41	109	39	61	31	71	33
Iron (mg)	6	47	9	50	5	45	6	43
Zinc (mg)	5	50	8	58	3	41	4	42
Copper (mg)	0.5	52	0.6	48	0.4	47	0.4	41
Sodium (mg)	1,313	45	1,630	42	930	38	957	35
Potassium (mg)	866	41	1,130	41	631	32	750	35

NOTE: When the CV is larger than 60 to 70 percent the distribution of daily intakes is nonnormal and the methods presented here are unreliable.
[a] Square root of the residual variance after accounting for subject, and sequence of observation (gender and age controlled by classifications).
[b] Nutrient intakes are for food only, data does not include intake from supplements.
[c] Folate reported in µg rather than as the new dietary folate equivalents (DFE).
SOURCE: Data from Continuing Survey of Food Intakes by Individuals 1994–1996.

Note that D/SD_D depends on the size of the difference between observed mean intake and the EAR and the standard deviation of that difference. For very large differences between observed mean intake and the EAR, it is likely that the ratio will exceed 1 and usual intake exceeds requirement. For smaller differences, the ability to critically interpret individual dietary intake data depends on the standard deviation of the difference between the observed intake

TABLE B-4 Estimates of Within-Subject Variation in Intake, Expressed as Standard Deviation (SD)[a] and Coefficient of Variation (CV) for Macronutrients and Cholesterol in Adults Aged 19 and Over

Nutrient[b]	Adults, Ages 19–50 y				Adults, Ages 51 y and Over			
	Females (n = 2,480)[c]		Males (n = 2,583)		Females (n = 2,162)		Males (n = 2,280)	
	SD	CV (%)	SD	CV (%)	SD	CV (%)	SD	CV (%)
Energy (kcal)	576	34	854	34	448	31	590	29
Fat (total, g)	29.9	48	42.7	44	24.0	45	31.8	42
Fat (saturated, g)	10.9	52	15.9	49	8.6	50	11.4	45
Fat (mono-unsaturated, g)	12.0	50	17.4	46	9.7	48	13.0	44
Fat (poly-unsaturated, g)	8.4	64	11.3	59	7.0	61	8.8	57
Carbohydrate (g)	75.2	35	109	35	59.9	32	79.5	32
Protein (g)	26.6	42	40.4	41	22.1	37	28.6	35
Fiber (g)	6.5	49	9.2	51	5.9	43	7.7	43
Cholesterol (mg)	168	77	227	66	144	70	201	66

NOTE: When the CV is larger than 60 to 70 percent the distribution of daily intakes is nonnormal and the methods presented here are unreliable.

[a] Square root of the residual variance after accounting for subject, and sequence of observation (gender and age controlled by classifications).

[b] Nutrient intakes are for food only, data does not include intake from supplements.

[c] Sample size was inadequate to provide separate estimates for pregnant or lactating women.

SOURCE: Data from Continuing Survey of Food Intakes by Individuals 1994–1996.

and the EAR. This standard deviation depends, among other factors, on the number of days of intake data that are available for the individual. The fewer days of intake data available for the individual, the larger the standard deviation of the difference (resulting in a smaller ratio D/SD_D) and the lower the likelihood of being able to assess adequacy or inadequacy.

Implementation of the Individual Assessment Approach

To implement the approach described above, the following information is needed:

TABLE B-5 Estimates of Within-Subject Variation in Intake, Expressed as Standard Deviation $(SD)^a$ and Coefficient of Variation (CV) for Macronutrients and Cholesterol in Adolescents and Children

Nutrient [b]	Adolescents Ages 9–18 y				Children Ages 4–8 y			
	Females (n = 1,002)		Males (n = 998)		Females (n = 817)		Males (n = 833)	
	SD	CV (%)	SD	CV (%)	SD	CV (%)	SD	CV (%)
Energy (kcal)	628	34	800	33	427	27	478	27
Fat (total, g)	29.8	45	38.2	42	21.3	37	23.9	37
Fat (saturated, g)	11.3	48	15.3	48	8.5	40	9.6	40
Fat (mono-unsaturated, g)	12.4	48	15.5	44	8.6	39	9.9	41
Fat (poly-unsaturated, g)	7.3	60	8.7	55	5.1	52	5.5	52
Carbohydrate (g)	88.1	35	113	35	61.7	29	70.8	30
Protein (g)	26.2	42	33.9	39	19.2	34	20.4	33
Fiber (g)	6.2	51	8.7	56	4.6	43	5.3	45
Cholesterol (mg)	145	72	199	71	129	70	137	66

NOTE: When the CV is larger than 60 to 70 percent the distribution of daily intakes is nonnormal and the methods presented here are unreliable.

[a] Square root of the residual variance after accounting for subject, and sequence of observation (gender and age controlled by classifications).

[b] Nutrient intakes are for food only, data does not include intake from supplements.

SOURCE: Data from Continuing Survey of Food Intakes by Individuals 1994–1996.

- $\bar{y}$, the mean of n days of intake for the individual;
- SD_{within}, the day-to-day standard deviation of the individual's intake for the nutrient;
- EAR, the median nutrient requirement; and
- SD_r, the standard deviation of requirements in the group.

For nutrients that do not have an EAR, this approach cannot be used. (Guidance on how to assess an individual's usual intake by comparing it to the Adequate Intake [AI] is provided later in this appendix.) When an EAR for the nutrient is provided in a DRI report, the standard deviation of requirements is also available in the form of a coefficient of variation of requirement or percentage of the EAR. In most cases, it is assumed to be 10 percent.

The day-to-day standard deviation in intakes is harder to determine because data that permit the calculation are scarce. Using data collected in the Beltsville One Year Dietary Survey (Mertz and Kelsay, 1984), Tarasuk and Beaton (1992) investigated intake patterns for several nutrients and produced estimates of, among other parameters, the day-to-day variance in intakes for those nutrients. Other estimates have been developed from research databases and from large survey data sets with replicate observations (e.g., the Continuing Survey of Food Intakes by Individuals [CSFII]). Tables B-2 through B-5 present pooled estimates of the day-to-day variance in intakes based on an analysis of the 1994–1996 CSFII data. Since a reliable estimate of the day-to-day variability in intakes for a specific individual is not typically available, the pooled estimates in Tables B-2 through B-5 should be used. This introduces other uncertainties, however.

Limitations of Using the EAR for Individual Assessment

The method described to compare an individual's observed intake to the EAR for the purpose of drawing conclusions about the usual intake of the individual cannot be implemented in all cases. Even when the appropriate calculations are carried out, incorrect conclusions may result if estimates of the SD of daily intake and the SD of requirements are incorrect. These two situations are discussed below.

The SD of Intake for the Individual Is Not Equal to the Pooled Estimate Obtained from CSFII or from the National Health and Nutrition Examination Survey

The value of the ratio D/SD_D critically depends on the SD of daily intake for the individual. It is recommended that the estimate obtained from CSFII (see Tables B-2 through B-5) be used for all individuals, even though it has been argued that the day-to-day variability in intakes is typically heterogeneous across individuals. Several researchers, including Tarasuk and Beaton (1992), have argued that day-to-day variability in intakes varies across individuals (see also Nusser et al., 1996); therefore a pooled variance estimate as suggested here might not be the optimal strategy. In theory, if many days of intake data Y_j were available for an individual, the within-individual variance in intakes could be computed in the standard manner:

$$V_{within} = \sum_j \left(Y_j = \bar{y} \right)^2 / (n-1)$$

where Y_j denotes the intake for the individual observed on the jth day and $\bar{y}$ is the mean of the n days of observed intakes. The within-individual standard deviation SD_{within} is computed as the square root of V_{within}. Unless a large number of nonconsecutive days (e.g., more than 10 or 12 days) of intake records are available for the individual, it is recommended that the pooled estimate from Tables B-2 through B-5 be used instead. Whereas this pooled estimate is likely to be incorrect for the individual, at this time there is no better alternative. More research is needed in this area that will permit estimating an adjustment of the pooled variance estimate to suit a particular individual.

The Day-To-Day Distribution of Intakes Is Not Normal

The assumption of normality (or near normality) of the observed intakes Y_j is critical, as the proposed approach relies on normality of the difference D. Normality of D will not be satisfied whenever the observed intakes Y_j (and consequently, the observed intake mean) are not normally distributed.

How does one decide whether the distribution of observed intakes for an individual is approximately normal? Typically there are not enough days of intake data available for an individual to be able to conduct a test of normality of the observed intakes. Therefore, one must rely on the CV of daily intakes that are presented in Tables B-2 through B-5.

As a rule, any nutrient with a CV above 60 to 70 percent should be considered to have a nonnormal distribution for the following reason: if daily intakes for an individual are normally distributed, then subtracting 2 SD of intake from the individual's mean should still result in a positive value, as intakes are restricted to being positive. Suppose that the CV of intake was 60 percent, then the SD of intake is $0.6 \times$ mean intake. If 2 SDs of intake are now subtracted from the individual's mean intake a negative value is obtained, indicating that the distribution of observed intakes around the individual's usual intake is not normal.

$$
\begin{aligned}
\text{Mean intake} - 2\ SD\ \text{intake} &= \text{mean intake} - 2 \times 0.6 \times \text{mean intake} \\
&= \text{mean intake} - 1.2\ \text{mean intake} \\
&= -0.2 \times \text{mean intake}.
\end{aligned}
$$

The value in the last equation is negative, suggesting that the normal model is not reasonable when the CV of intake is above 60 to 70 percent.

Data presented in Tables B-2 through B-5 indicate that it is not possible to use this approach to assess the adequacy of vitamin A, vitamin C, vitamin E, and some other nutrients. In these cases, the distribution of daily intakes cannot be assumed to be normal, and thus observed daily intake cannot be used to carry out the assessment.

Because the distributions of daily intake for many nutrients are nonnormal, more research is needed in order to extend this methodology to all nutrients of interest.

Requirement Distribution Is Not Normal

The proposed approach relies also on normality of the requirement distribution. When requirements are not distributed in a symmetrical, approximately normal fashion around the EAR, results may be biased. For example, the confidence with which it can be concluded that intake is adequate may be less than 85 percent even though the observed ratio D/SD_D is equal to 1.

Iron is an example of a nutrient for which the distribution of requirements is not normal. Iron requirements in menstruating women are skewed, with a long tail to the right. In this situation, the method described above does not produce reliable results. No alternative can be offered at this time; more research is needed in this area.

Incorrect Specification of the SD of Requirement

Until now, little if any attention has been paid to reliably estimating the variance of nutrient requirement distributions. DRI reports (IOM, 1997, 1998b, 2000) have assumed that the *CV* of requirements for most nutrients is 10 percent of the EAR, unless other information is known (e.g., niacin is given as 15 percent). Given an EAR and a *CV* of requirement, an *SD* of requirement can be calculated as $SD_r = CV \times EAR$. For example, if the EAR of a nutrient is 120 units/day and the *CV* of requirement is 10 percent, then the *SD* of requirement will be $0.1 \times 120 = 12$ units/day.

It is not clear that the fixed 10 percent (or 15 percent) *CV* estimates across nutrients result in reliable estimators of the *SD* of requirement. Since the *SD* of requirement is an important component of the *SD* of *D*, an inaccurate value of SD_r will result in an inaccurate value of SD_D and hence an inaccurate value of the ratio D/SD_D.

At this time, no better alternatives than using the *CV* of the requirement as given in the DRI reports have been identified, and thus the results of such analyses should be interpreted with caution.

INDIVIDUAL ASSESSMENT FOR NUTRIENTS WITH AN AI

Before discussing a statistical approach to individual assessment for nutrients with an Adequate Intake (AI) instead of an Estimated Average Requirement (EAR), it is critical to emphasize the difference between these two Dietary Reference Intakes (DRIs). The EAR represents the median nutrient requirement of a given life stage and gender group, and by definition, an intake at the level of the EAR will be inadequate for half the group. In contrast, the AI represents an intake that is likely to exceed the actual requirements of almost all healthy individuals in a life stage and gender group. In this respect it is analogous to the Recommended Dietary Allowance (RDA); however, because of the imprecise nature of the data used to establish AIs, it may often be higher than an RDA would be if appropriate data were available to calculate one.

The approach discussed previously to assess nutrient adequacy compares an individual's intake to the EAR, and considers variability in both intake and requirement when determining how confident one can be in concluding that intake is adequate. In other words, intakes are compared to *median requirements*. In the case of the AI, however, intakes are compared to an intake value already *in excess* of the median requirement, perhaps by a very large margin. Thus, when intakes are compared to the AI, all one can truly conclude is whether intake is above the AI or not. Although an intake that is statistically above the AI is certainly adequate, intakes below the AI are also likely to be adequate for a considerable proportion of individuals. Thus, great caution must be exercised when interpreting intakes relative to AIs.

How can individual assessment be carried out when the nutrient of interest does not have an EAR? Using calcium as an example, one is limited to comparing the individual's *usual* intake to the AI. The conclusions that can be drawn from such a comparison are rather narrow: if the usual intake is determined with desired accuracy to be larger than the AI, then the individual's usual intake of the nutrient is likely to be adequate. The converse, however, is not true. At the desired level of confidence, nothing can be concluded from the analysis if it is found that the individual's usual intake is *not* larger than the AI.

A simple z-test to decide whether an individual's unobservable usual intake is larger than the AI can be used. The test assumes that daily intakes for an individual have a distribution that is approximately normal around the individual's usual intake. The *SD* of daily intake is necessary to carry out the test. Because large numbers of daily intakes for an individual are typically not available to reliably estimate the day-to-day variability, the pooled day-to-day *SD* of intake from CSFII (see Tables B-2 through B-5) or from NHANES is used.

The *z*-statistic is constructed as follows:

$$z = \sqrt{n} \times (\text{observed mean intake} - \text{AI}) / SD \text{ of daily intake.}$$

By rearrangement, this can also be expressed as:

$$z = (\text{observed mean intake} - \text{AI}) / (SD \text{ of daily intake} / \sqrt{n}).$$

The *z*-statistic is then compared to tabulated values (a selection of which are presented in Table B-6), to decide whether the desired level of accuracy is achieved when stating that the usual intake is larger than the AI.

For example, consider a nutrient such as calcium with an AI of 1,000 mg /day, and suppose that the *SD* of daily intake from CSFII for the appropriate life stage and gender group is 325 mg/day.

TABLE B-6 Selected Values of *z* and the Associated Level of Confidence When Concluding That Individual Usual Intake Is Larger Than the Adequate Intake (AI) or Less Than the Tolerable Upper Intake Level (UL)

Criterion	Conclusion	Probability of Correct Conclusion	
$z > 2.00$	Usual intake is adequate (excessive)	0.98	
$z > 1.65$	Usual intake is adequate (excessive)	0.95	
$z > 1.50$	Usual intake is adequate (excessive)	0.93	
$z > 1.25$	Usual intake is adequate (excessive)	0.90	
$z > 1.00$	Usual intake is adequate (excessive)	0.85	
$z > 0.85$	Usual intake is adequate (excessive)	0.80	
$z > 0.68$	Usual intake is adequate (excessive)	0.75	
$z > 0.50$	Usual intake is adequate (excessive)	0.70	
$z > 0.00$	Usual intake is adequate (excessive/safe)	0.50	
$z > -0.50$	Usual intake is adequate (excessive)	0.30	(0.70 probability usual intake is safe)
$z > -0.85$	Usual intake is adequate (excessive)	0.20	(0.80 probability usual intake is safe)
$z > -1.00$	Usual intake is adequate (excessive)	0.15	(0.85 probability usual intake is safe)

SOURCE: Adapted from Snedecor and Cochran (1980).

Given five individuals, each with three days of intake records and observed mean intakes of 1,050, 1,100, 1,150, 1,200, and 1,250 mg/day, respectively, what can be determined about the adequacy of their usual intakes? Assume that, to determine if the usual intake is higher than the AI, a minimum confidence level of 85 percent is desired.

To calculate the z-values for each of the five individuals, first divide the SD of daily intake by the $\sqrt{3}$ (as 3 daily records are available for each). In this example, $325/\sqrt{3}$ equals 188. The z-values are now computed as (observed mean intake − AI)/188. For the five individuals, the corresponding z-values are 0.27, 0.53, 0.80, 1.07, and 1.33, respectively. From a standard z-table the probabilities of correctly concluding that the usual intake is larger than the AI for each of the five individuals are 61, 70, 79, 86, and 91 percent, respectively. Only for the last two individuals, with observed mean intakes of 1,200 and 1,250 mg /day, would there be an 85 percent confidence level when stating that usual intakes are greater than 1,000 mg/day.

The value of the z-statistic will increase whenever

- the difference between the observed mean intake and the AI increases;
- the SD of daily intake for the nutrient is low; and
- the number of days of intake data available for the individual increases.

This z-test relies on the assumption of normality of daily intakes. For nutrients such as vitamin A, vitamin B_{12}, and others with a CV of daily intake larger than 60 to 70 percent, this test is likely to perform poorly. While the calculations are still possible, the level of assurance resulting from the test will be incorrect. The performance of the test also depends on accurately estimating the day-to-day variability in intakes for the individual. It is suggested that the pooled SD of daily intake obtained, for example, from Tables B-2 through B-5 be used in the calculations even though it is likely to be a poor estimate of the individual's true day-to-day variability in intakes. As stated earlier, a more justifiable alternative cannot be offered at this time, as no extensive studies on the dependence of individual SD of intake and individual mean intake have been published. More research is needed in this area.

ASSESSING EXCESSIVE INTAKE AT THE
INDIVIDUAL LEVEL

Evaluation of the adequacy of an individual's usual intake of a nutrient has been discussed. Since food fortification is now commonplace and supplement intake is also on the rise, it is important to evaluate whether an individual's usual intake of a nutrient might be excessive. To decide whether an individual has chronic consumption of a nutrient at levels that may increase the risk of adverse effects, the *usual* nutrient intake is compared to the Tolerable Upper Intake Level (UL) established for the nutrient.

Because *usual* intakes are unobservable, the uncertainty of how well observed mean intake estimates usual intake must be accounted for, similar to comparing intake to the Adequate Intake (AI) as discussed in the previous section. In this case, however, the z-statistic is constructed by subtracting the UL from the observed mean intake, and dividing the difference by the *SD* of daily intake over the square root of the number of days of intake available for the individual.

$$z = (\text{observed mean intake} - \text{UL})/(SD \text{ of daily intake}/\sqrt{n})$$

The resulting z-statistic is compared to tabulated values (Table B-6), and the confidence level associated with the conclusion that the usual intake is below the UL is obtained. If the resulting confidence level is at least as high as the desired level, then it can be concluded that the individual's usual intake of the nutrient is below the UL and thus a tolerable level of intake for the individual. If the resulting confidence level is not as high as the desired level, then it cannot be conclusively stated that intake is risk free.

Caution also applies in this case. The z-test performs well when daily intakes are approximately normally distributed, but may give incorrect confidence levels when the distribution of daily intakes departs from the normal. The *SD* of daily intake should accurately reflect the day-to-day variability in intakes for the individual. In the absence of better information about individual *SD* of daily intake, it is recommended that the pooled estimate of the SD of intake computed from a large nationwide food consumption survey be used. Use of this pooled estimate of the *SD* of daily intakes is not ideal for the individual, but a reliable alternative is not available at this time.

In the case of regular supplement users, an overestimate of the individual day-to-day variability of intakes may result. If the day-to-day variability for a supplement user were smaller, then the z-statistic obtained from the assessment would be an underestimate.

When using the proposed method it is important to note that the pooled estimates of the within-person standard deviation of intakes in Tables B-2 to B-5 are based on data on nutrients from food only, not food plus supplements. This suggests the need for caution in using these estimates in assessing individual intakes relative to the UL. For some nutrients, ULs are defined on the basis of total intake (food plus supplements), and the estimates of the within-person standard deviation of intakes based on food alone may not be the same as those based on food plus supplements. For other nutrients, ULs refer only to nutrient intake from food fortificants, supplements, and pharmacological products. In these cases, the proposed methods are even less reliable, as currently there are no estimates of the within-person standard deviation of intakes from supplement use alone.

C

Assessing Prevalence of Inadequate Intakes for Groups: Statistical Foundations

This appendix provides the formal statistical justification for the methods for assessing the prevalence of inadequate intakes that were described in Chapter 4. Additional details can be found in Carriquiry (1999).

Let Y_{ij} denote the observed intake of a dietary component on the jth day for the ith individual in the sample, and define $y_i = E\{Y_{ij} \mid i\}$ to be that individual's usual intake of the component. Further, let r_i denote the requirement of the dietary component for the ith individual. Conceptually, because day-to-day variability in requirements is typically present, r_i is defined as $= E\{R_{ij} \mid i\}$ and, as in the case of intakes, R_{ij} denotes the (often unobserved) daily requirement of the dietary component for the ith individual on the jth day. In the remainder of this appendix, usual intakes and usual requirements are simply referred to as intakes and requirements, respectively.

The problem of interest is assessing the proportion of individuals in the group with inadequate intake of the dietary component. The term inadequate means that the individual's usual intake is not meeting that individual's requirement.

THE JOINT DISTRIBUTION OF INTAKE AND REQUIREMENT

Let $F_{Y,R}(y,r)$ denote the joint distribution of intakes and requirements, and let $f_{Y,R}(y,r)$ be the corresponding density. If $f_{Y,R}(y,r)$ (or a reliable density estimate) is available, then

$$\text{Pr(nutrient inadequacy)} = \text{Pr}(y < r)$$

$$= \int_0^\infty \int_0^r f_{Y,R}(t, s)\,ds\,dt. \tag{1}$$

For a given estimate of the joint distribution $f_{Y,R}$, obtaining equation 1 is trivial. The problem is not the actual probability calculation but rather the estimation of the joint distribution of intakes and requirements in the population.

To reduce the data burden for estimating $f_{Y,R}$, approaches such as the probability approach proposed by the National Research Council (NRC, 1986) and the Estimated Average Requirement (EAR) cut-point method proposed by Beaton (1994), make an implicit assumption that intakes and requirements are independent random variables—that what an individual consumes of a nutrient is not correlated with that individual's requirement for the nutrient. If the assumption of independence holds, then the joint distribution of intakes and requirements can be factorized into the product of the two marginal densities as follows:

$$f_{Y,R}(r, y) = f_R(r)f_Y(y) \tag{2}$$

where $f_Y(y)$ and $f_R(r)$ are the marginal densities of usual intakes of the nutrient, and of requirements respectively, in the population of interest.

Note that under the formulation in equation 2, the problem of assessing prevalence of nutrient inadequacy becomes tractable. Indeed, methods for reliable estimation of $f_Y(y)$ have been proposed (e.g., Guenther et al., 1997; Nusser et al., 1996) and data are abundant. Estimating $f_R(r)$ is still problematic because requirement data are scarce for most nutrients, but the mean (or perhaps the median) and the variance of $f_R(r)$ can often be computed with some degree of reliability (Beaton, 1999; Beaton and Chery, 1988; Dewey et al., 1996; FAO/WHO, 1988; FAO/WHO/UNU, 1985). Approaches for combining $f_R(r)$ and $f_Y(y)$ for prevalence assessments that require different amounts of information (and assumptions) about the unknown requirement density $f_R(r)$ and the joint distribution $F_{Y,R}(y, r)$ are discussed next.

THE PROBABILITY APPROACH

The probability approach to estimating the prevalence of nutrient inadequacy was proposed by the National Research Council (NRC, 1986). The idea is simple. For a given a distribution of requirements in the population, the first step is to compute a risk curve that associates intake levels with risk levels under the assumed requirement distribution.

Formally, the risk curve[1] is obtained from the cumulative distribution function (*cdf*) of requirements. If we let $F_R(.)$ denote the *cdf* of the requirements of a dietary component in the population, then

$$F_R(a) = \Pr(\text{requirements} \leq a)$$

for any positive value *a*. Thus, the *cdf* F_R takes on values between 0 and 1. The risk curve ρ (.) is defined as

$$\rho(a) = 1 - F_R(a) = 1 - \Pr(\text{requirements} \leq a)$$

A simulated example of a risk curve is given in Figure 4-3. This risk curve is easy to read. On the *x*-axis the values correspond to intake levels. On the *y*-axis the values correspond to the risk of nutrient inadequacy given a certain intake level. Rougher assessments are also possible. For a given range of intake values, the associated risk can be estimated as the risk value that corresponds to the midpoint of the range.

For assumed requirement distributions with usual intake distributions estimated from dietary survey data, how should the risk curves be combined?

It seems intuitively appealing to argue as follows. Consider again the simulated risk curve in Figure 4-3 and suppose the usual intake distribution for this simulated nutrient in a population has been estimated. If that estimated usual intake distribution places a very high probability on intake values less than 90, then one would con-

---

[1] When the distribution of requirements is approximately normal, the *cdf* can be easily evaluated in the usual way for any intake level *a*. Let *z* represent the standardized intake, computed as $z = (a - \text{mean requirement}) / SD$, where *SD* denotes the standard deviation of requirement. Values of $F_{R(z)}$ can be found in most statistical textbooks, or more importantly, are given by most, if not all, statistical software packages. For example, in SAS, the function probnorm(*b*) evaluates the standard normal *cdf* at a value *b*. Thus, the "drawing the risk curve" is a conceptualization rather than a practical necessity.

clude that most individuals in the group are likely to have inadequate intake of the nutrient. If, on the other hand, the usual nutrient intake distribution places a very high probability on intakes above 90, then one would be confident that only a small fraction of the population is likely to have inadequate intake. Illustrations of these two extreme cases are given in Figures 4-4 and 4-5.

In general, one would expect that the usual intake distribution and the risk curve for a nutrient show some overlap, as in Figure 4-6. In this case, estimating the portion of individuals likely to have inadequate intakes is equivalent to computing a weighted average of risk, as explained below.

The quantity of interest is not the risk associated with a certain intake level but rather the *expected risk of inadequacy* in the population. This expectation is based on the usual intake distribution for the nutrient in the population. In other words, prevalence of nutrient inadequacy is defined as the expected risk for the distribution of intakes in the population. To derive the estimate of prevalence, we first define

• $p(y)$ as the probability, under the usual intake distribution, associated with each intake level y and
• $\rho(y)$ as the risk calculated from the requirement distribution. The calculation of prevalence is simple

$$\text{Prevalence} = \sum_{y=0}^{\infty} \rho(y)p(y) \tag{3}$$

where, in practice, the sum is carried out only to intake levels where the risk of inadequacy becomes about zero.

Notice that equation 3 is simply a weighted average of risk values, where the weights are given by the probabilities of observing the intakes associated with those risks. Formally, the expected risk is given by

$$E\{\text{risk}\} = \int_0^\infty \rho(y)dF$$
$$= \int_0^\infty \rho(y)f(y)dy$$

where $\rho(y)$ denotes the risk value for an intake level y, F is the usual intake distribution, and $f(y)$ is the value of the usual intake density at intake level y.

When the NRC proposed the probability approach in 1986, statistical software and personal computers were not as commonplace as they are today. The NRC included a program in the report that could be used to estimate the prevalence of nutrient inadequacy using the probability approach. As an illustration, the NRC also mentioned a simple computational method: rather than adding up many products $\rho(y)\, p(y)$ associated with different values of intakes, intakes are grouped by constructing m bins. The estimated probabilities associated with each bin are simply the frequencies of intakes in the population that "fall into" each bin. (These frequencies are determined by the usual intake distribution in the population.) The average risk associated with intakes in a bin is approximated as the risk associated with the midpoint of the bin. An example of this computation is given on page 28, Table 5-1, of the NRC report (1986). Currently, implementation of the probability approach can be carried out with standard software (such as BMDP, SAS, Splus, SPSS, etc.).

In general, researchers assume that requirement distributions are normal, with mean and variance as estimated from experimental data. Even under normality, however, an error in the estimation of either the mean or the variance (or both) of the requirement distribution may lead to biased prevalence estimates. NRC (1986) provides various examples of the effect of changing the mean and the variance of the requirement distribution on prevalence estimates. Although the probability approach was highly sensitive to specification of the mean requirement, it appeared to be relatively insensitive to other parameters of the distribution as long as the final distribution approximated symmetry. Thus, although the shape of the requirement distribution is clearly an important component when using the probability approach to estimate the prevalence of nutrient inadequacy, the method appears to be robust to errors in shape specifications.

The NRC report discusses the effect of incorrectly specifying the form of the requirement distribution on the performance of the probability approach to assess prevalence (see pages 32–33 of the 1986 NRC report), but more research is needed in this area, particularly on nonsymmetrical distributions. Statistical theory dictates that the use of the incorrect probability model is likely to result in an inaccurate estimate of prevalence except in special cases. The pioneering efforts of the 1986 NRC committee need to be continued to assess the extent to which an incorrect model specification may affect the properties of prevalence estimates.

THE EAR CUT-POINT METHOD

The probability approach described in the previous section is simple to apply and provides unbiased and consistent estimates of the prevalence of nutrient inadequacy under relatively mild conditions (i.e., intake and requirement are independent, distribution of requirement is known). In fact, if intakes and requirements are independent and if the distributions of intakes and requirements are known, the probability approach results in optimal (in the sense of mean squared error) estimates of the prevalence of nutrient inadequacy in a group. However, application of the probability approach requires the user to choose a probability model (a probability distribution) for requirements in the group. Estimating a density is a challenging problem in the best of cases; when data are scare, it may be difficult to decide, for example, whether a normal model or a t model may be a more appropriate representation of the distribution of requirements in the group. The difference between these two probability models lies in the tails of the distribution; both models may be centered at the same median and both reflect symmetry around the median, but in the case of t with few degrees of freedom, the tails are heavier, and thus one would expect to see more extreme values under the t model than under the normal model. Would using the normal model to construct the risk curve affect the prevalence of inadequacy when requirements are really distributed as t random variables? This is a difficult question to answer. When it is not clear whether a certain probability model best represents the requirements in the population, a good alternative might be to use a method that is less parametric, that is, that requires milder assumptions on the t model itself. The Estimated Average Requirement (EAR) cut-point method, a less parametric version of the probability approach, may sometimes provide a simple, effective way to estimate the prevalence of nutrient inadequacy in the group even when the underlying probability model is difficult to determine precisely. The only feature of the shape of the underlying model that is required for good performance of the cut-point method is symmetry; in the example above, both the normal and the t models would satisfy the less demanding symmetry requirement and therefore choosing between one or the other becomes an unnecessary step.

The cut-point method is very simple: estimate prevalence of inadequate intakes as the proportion of the population with usual intakes below the median requirement (EAR).

To understand how the cut-point method works, the reader is referred to Chapter 4, where the joint distribution of intakes and requirements is defined. Figure 4-8 shows a simulated joint distribution of intakes and requirements. To generate the joint distribution, usual intakes and requirements for 3,000 individuals were simulated from a χ^2 distribution with 7 degrees of freedom and a normal distribution, respectively. Intakes and requirements were generated as independent random variables. The usual intake distribution was rescaled to have a mean of 1,600 and standard deviation of 400. The normal distribution used to represent requirements had a mean of 1,200 and standard deviation of 200. Note that intakes and requirements are uncorrelated (and in this example, independent) and that the usual intake distribution is skewed. An individual whose intake is below the *mean requirement* does not necessarily have an inadequate intake.

Because inferences are based on joint rather than the univariate distributions, an individual consuming a nutrient at a level below the mean of the population requirement may be satisfying the individual's own requirements. That is the case for all the individuals represented in Figure 4-8 by points that appear below the 45° line and to the left of the vertical EAR reference line, in triangular area B.

To estimate prevalence, proceed as in equation 1, or equivalently, count the points that appear above the 45° line (the shaded area), because for them $y < r$. This is not a practical method because typically information needed for estimating the joint distribution is not available. Can this proportion be approximated in some other way? The probability approach in the previous section is one such approximation. The EAR cut-point method is a shortcut to the probability approach and provides another approximation to the true prevalence of inadequacy.

When certain assumptions hold, the number of individuals with intakes to the left of the vertical intake = EAR line is more or less the same as the number of individuals over the 45° line. That is,

$$\int_0^\infty \int_0^r f(y, r)\,dy\,dr \approx \int_0^a f(y)\,dy$$

or equivalently,

$$\Pr\{y \le r\} \approx F_r(a)$$

where $F_y(a) = \mathrm{PR}\{y \le a\}$ is the *cdf* of intakes evaluated at a, for $a = EAR$. In fact, it is easy to show that when $E(r) = E(y)$:

$$\Pr(y \le r) = F_Y(EAR)$$

The prevalence of inadequate intakes can be assessed as long as one has an estimate of the usual nutrient intake distribution (which is almost always available) and of the median requirement in the population, or EAR, which can be obtained reliably from relatively small experiments.

The quantile $F_Y(EAR)$ is an approximately unbiased estimator of $\Pr\{y \le r\}$ if

• $f_{Y,R}(y,r) = f_Y(y) \, f_R(r)$, that is intakes and requirements are independent random variables.
• $\Pr\{r \le -\alpha\} = \Pr\{r \ge \alpha\}$ for any $\alpha > 0$, that is, the distribution of requirements is symmetrical around its mean; and
• $\sigma_r^2 > \sigma_y^2$, where σ_r^2 and σ_y^2 denote the variance of the distribution of requirements and of intakes, respectively.

When any of the conditions above are not satisfied, $F_Y(EAR) \ne \Pr\{y \le r\}$, in general. Whether $F_Y(EAR)$ is biased upward or downward depends on factors such as the relative sizes of the mean intake and the EAR.

D

Assessing the Performance of the EAR Cut-Point Method for Estimating Prevalence

This appendix presents the results of preliminary computer simulations evaluating the performance of the Estimated Average Requirement (EAR) cut-point method for estimating the prevalence of nutrient inadequacy. The simulations provide information on the performance of this model when its key assumptions are violated.

INTRODUCTION

In Chapter 4, an approach to estimating the prevalence of inadequate intakes in a group, called the Estimated Average Requirement (EAR) cut-point method, was introduced. This method is a short-cut of the probability approach for assessing nutrient inadequacy that was proposed by the National Research Council (NRC, 1986), and discussed in Appendix C of this report.

As stated in Chapter 4, the EAR cut-point method produces reliable estimates of the proportion of individuals in a group whose usual intakes do not meet their requirements, as long as the following assumptions hold:

- intakes and requirements of the nutrient are independent;
- the distribution of requirements in the group is symmetrical about the EAR; and
- the variance of the distribution of requirements is smaller than the variance of the distribution of usual intakes.

A reliable estimate of the distribution of usual intakes in the group is also needed in order to estimate the prevalence of inadequacy.

In addition, it was stated that the estimates of inadequacy would be essentially unbiased when the actual prevalence of inadequacy in the group is close to 50 percent. As the true prevalence approaches 0 or 100 percent, the performance of the EAR cut-point method declines, even if the conditions listed above are met.

To test the EAR cut-point method, some preliminary simulation studies were performed. The reliability of this method of estimating the prevalence of inadequacy was evaluated in cases where the assumptions above were met, and also in cases in which one or more of the assumptions were violated. For example, the EAR cut-point method was used to evaluate groups in which (1) intakes and requirements were correlated (for example, food energy), (2) the standard deviation of requirements (SD_r) was larger than the standard deviation of usual intakes (SD_i), and (3) the distribution of requirements was skewed (as is the case of iron in menstruating women).

This appendix does not test the performance of the probability approach. The probability approach, by construction, will perform well whenever intakes and requirements are independent, and whenever the form of the distribution of requirements is known. As in the EAR cut-point method, a reliable estimate of the distribution of usual intakes in the group must be available to ensure an unbiased estimate of the prevalence of inadequacy in the group.

Results of the simulation studies are reported in three sections. The first section examines the impact of violating the independence assumption on the estimates of prevalence. In the second section, the robustness of the EAR cut-point method to departures from the assumption of small SD_r relative to SD_i is tested. Finally, in the third section, the effects of departures from the assumption of a symmetrical requirement distribution are considered. In each section, a description of how the simulations were run is followed by a summary of the major findings. The simulation studies presented are preliminary and by no means definitive. They are intended to provide initial insight into the performance of this short-cut of the probability approach for estimating inadequacy. It is hoped that this report will encourage other researchers to proceed from the information presented here and conduct further research on this important topic.

INTAKES AND REQUIREMENTS ARE CORRELATED

The impact of violating the assumption of independence between intakes and requirements was evaluated by estimating prevalence of inadequacy in a group in which the correlation varied from 0 through 1. The intakes and requirements for the group were generated from a bivariate normal distribution in which the mean and standard deviation of usual intake were fixed at 90 and 30 units, respectively. Several cases were considered for the distribution of requirements. The Estimated Average Requirement (EAR) was fixed at three values: 55, 70, and 90 units, and the SD_r was also set at three values: 7.5, 15, and 30 units. Thus, the effect of increasing the correlation between intake and requirement for nine different scenarios for the joint distribution of intakes and requirements was investigated. It is important to point out that neither the probability approach nor its shortcut, the EAR cut-point method require that the distribution of usual intakes in the group be normal. The performance of either method does not depend in any way on the shape of the distribution of usual intakes in the group. Intakes from a normal distribution were generated only for convenience.

In each case, the *true* prevalence was obtained as the proportion of individuals whose usual intakes were below their requirements for the nutrient in a population of 50,000. From this population, smaller groups of 2,000 were sampled 200 times. The *estimated* prevalence was obtained as the proportion of individuals whose usual intakes were below the corresponding EAR (i.e., by application of the EAR cut-point method) in each of the 200 groups. The estimates of prevalence presented here are the means, over the 200 replicates, of the estimates of prevalence in each of the groups.

In Figures D-1 through D-9, the solid lines and dots represent the *true* prevalence at each value of the correlation between intakes and requirements. The dashed lines and squares represent the average estimates of prevalence (over the 200 replicates) at each correlation value between intakes and requirements.

Box D-1 *Major findings—Intakes and requirements are correlated*

• When the SD_r is small relative to the SD_i, no serious biases on the estimate of prevalence are evident even at correlation values as high as 0.5 or 0.6 (Figures D-1 and D-4).

• When the SD_r increases relative to the SD_i, increasing the correlation between intakes and requirements can result in noticeable biases in the prevalence of inadequacy even when the correlation is no larger than about 0.4 (Figures D-2 and D-5).

• When the SD_r is as large as the SD_i, the bias in the estimate of prevalence can be significant even if the correlation between intakes and requirements is 0. This indicates that the EAR cut-point method is less robust to departures from the last assumption (variance of requirements must be smaller than variance of usual intake) (Figures D-3 and D-6).

• When mean intake is equal to the EAR (prevalence is exactly equal to 50 percent), neither increasing the correlation coefficient to 1 nor equating the variances of requirements and intakes introduces a bias in the estimated prevalence (Figures D-7, D-8, and D-9).

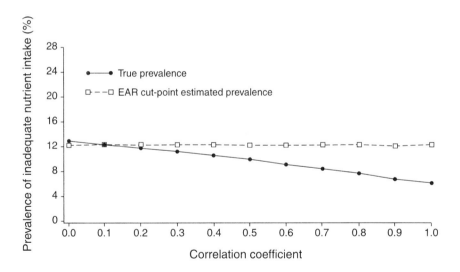

FIGURE D-1 The effect of correlation between usual intake and requirement on the prevalence of inadequate intakes estimated using the Estimated Average Requirement (EAR) cut-point method for 10 values of the correlation. For all correlations, mean intake = 90, standard deviation (*SD*) of intake = 30, EAR = 55, and *SD* of requirement = 7.5 units.

NOTE: When the *SD* of requirement is small relative to the *SD* of intake, there is no serious bias of the EAR cut-point method until correlation reaches 0.5 to 0.6.

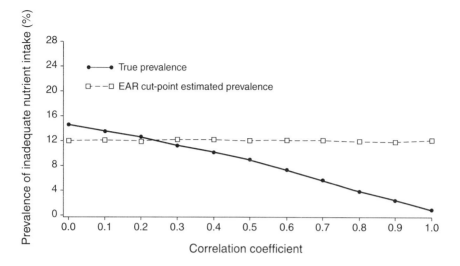

FIGURE D-2 The effect of correlation between usual intake and requirement on the prevalence of inadequate intakes estimated using the Estimated Average Requirement (EAR) cut-point method for 10 values of the correlation. For all correlations, mean intake = 90, standard deviation (*SD*) of intake = 30, EAR = 55, and *SD* of requirement = 15 units.

NOTE: When the *SD* of requirement increases relative to the *SD* of intake, increasing the correlation between intake and requirements can result in noticeable bias of the EAR cut-point method even when the correlation is as low as 0.4.

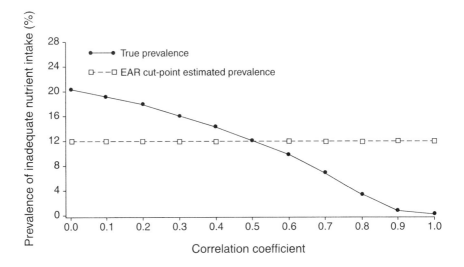

FIGURE D-3 The effect of correlation between usual intake and requirement on the prevalence of inadequate intakes estimated using the Estimated Average Requirement (EAR) cut-point method for 10 values of the correlation. For all correlations, mean intake = 90, standard deviation (*SD*) of intake = 30, EAR = 55, and *SD* of requirement = 30 units.

NOTE: When the *SD* of requirement is as large as the *SD* of intake, the estimate of prevalence of inadequate intakes using the EAR cut-point method shows significant bias even when the correlation between intake and requirement is zero.

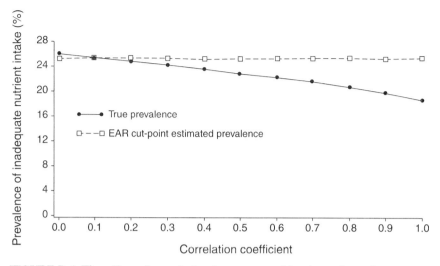

FIGURE D-4 The effect of correlation between usual intake and requirement on the prevalence of inadequate intakes estimated using the Estimated Average Requirement (EAR) cut-point method for 10 values of the correlation. For all correlations, mean intake = 90, standard deviation *(SD)* of intake = 30, EAR = 70, and *SD* of requirement = 7.5 units.

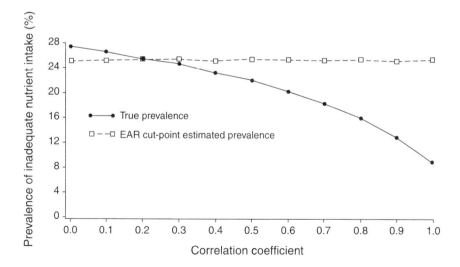

FIGURE D-5 The effect of correlation between usual intake and requirement on the prevalence of inadequate intakes estimated using the Estimated Average Requirement (EAR) cut-point method for 10 values of the correlation. For all correlations, mean intake = 90, standard deviation *(SD)* of intake = 30, EAR = 70, and *SD* of requirement = 15 units.

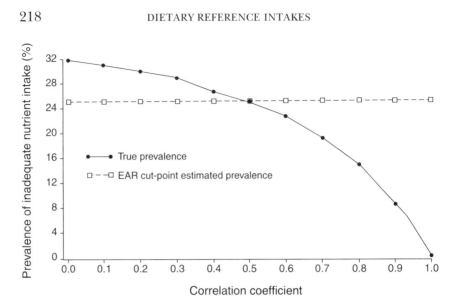

FIGURE D-6 The effect of correlation between usual intake and requirement on the prevalence of inadequate intakes estimated using the Estimated Average Requirement (EAR) cut-point method for 10 values of the correlation. For all correlations, mean intake = 90, standard deviation *(SD)* of intake = 30, EAR = 70, and *SD* of requirement = 30 units.

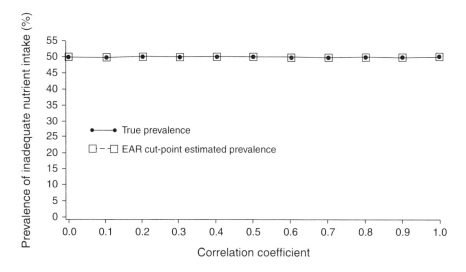

FIGURE D-7 The effect of correlation between usual intake and requirement on the prevalence of inadequate intakes estimated using the Estimated Average Requirement (EAR) cut-point method for 10 values of the correlation. For all correlations, mean intake = 90, standard deviation (*SD*) of intake = 30, EAR = 90, and *SD* of requirement = 7.5 units.

NOTE: When mean intake is equal to the EAR (prevalence of inadequate intakes is 50 percent), increasing the correlation between intake and requirement introduces no bias in the prevalence estimate using the EAR cut-point method.

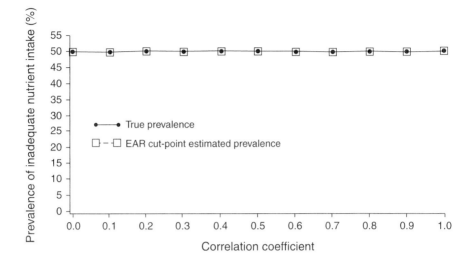

FIGURE D-8 The effect of correlation between usual intake and requirement on the prevalence of inadequate intakes estimated using the Estimated Average Requirement (EAR) cut-point method for 10 values of the correlation. For all correlations, mean intake = 90, standard deviation (*SD*) of intake = 30, EAR = 90, and *SD* of requirement = 15 units.

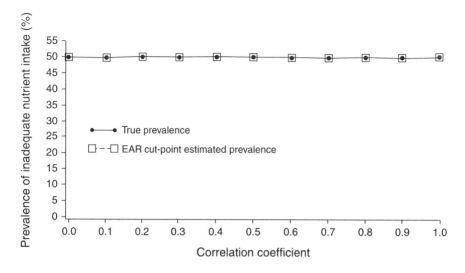

FIGURE D-9 The effect of correlation between usual intake and requirement on the prevalence of inadequate intakes estimated using the Estimated Average Requirement (EAR) cut-point method for 10 values of the correlation. For all correlations, mean intake = 90, standard deviation (*SD*) of intake = 30, EAR = 90, and *SD* of requirement = 30 units.

NOTE: When mean intake is equal to the EAR (prevalence of inadequate intakes is 50 percent), a variance of requirement as large as the variance of intake introduces no bias in the prevalence estimate using the EAR cut-point method.

Figures D-10, D-11, and D-12 show the bias of the prevalence estimates obtained from application of the EAR cut-point method relative to the true prevalence. The bias is calculated as the difference between the average prevalence estimate over the 200 replicates, and the true prevalence in the group. These three figures summarize the results presented in Figures D-1 through D-9.

In Figure D-10 the solid line and dots represents the bias in the estimated prevalence at various levels of the correlation between intakes and requirements for the case where the EAR is 55 units and the SD_r is 7.5. The dotted line and squares represents the bias of the EAR cut-point prevalence estimate when the SD_r is increased to 15 units. Finally, the dashed line and stars shows the amount of bias in the EAR cut-point prevalence estimates when the SD_r is equal to the SD_i of 30 units. Notice that when SD_r is small, the bias in the prevalence estimate is small, even at very high values of the correla-

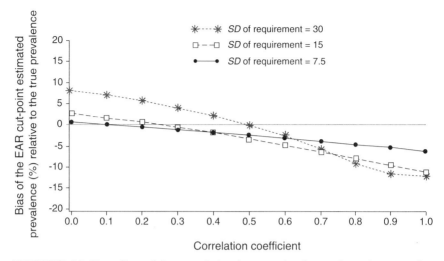

FIGURE D-10 The effect of the correlation between intakes and requirements for 10 values of the correlation on the bias of the estimated prevalence using the Estimated Average Requirement (EAR) cut-point method. For all correlations, mean intake = 90, standard deviation (*SD*) of intake = 30, and EAR = 55. The *SD* of requirement was set to 7.5 units (solid line with dots), 15 units (dashed lines with squares), and 30 units (dotted line with stars).

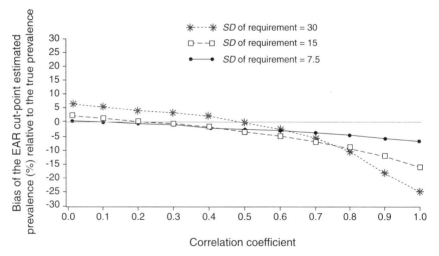

FIGURE D-11 The effect of correlation between intakes and requirements on the bias of the estimated prevalence using the Estimated Average Requirement (EAR) cut-point method for 10 values of the correlation. For all correlations, mean intake = 90, standard deviation (*SD*) of intake = 30, and EAR = 70. The *SD* of requirement was set to 7.5 units (solid line with dots), 15 units (dashed lines with squares), and 30 units (dotted line with stars).

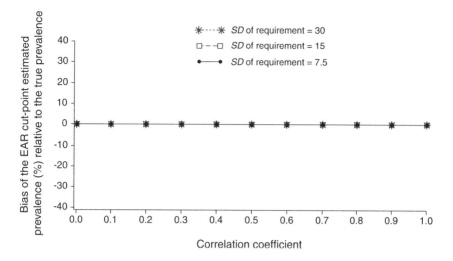

FIGURE D-12 The effect of correlation between intakes and requirements on the bias of the estimated prevalence using the Estimated Average Requirement (EAR) cut-point method for 10 values of the correlation. For all correlations, mean intake = 90, standard deviation (*SD*) of intake = 30, and EAR = 90. The *SD* of requirement was set to 7.5 units (solid line with dots), 15 units (dashed lines with squares), and 30 units (dotted line with stars).

NOTE: When the true prevalence of inadequacy is 50 percent (mean intake equals the EAR) neither increasing the correlation between intake and requirement or increasing the *SD* of requirement relative to the *SD* of intake introduces any bias of the prevalence estimate.

tion coefficient. The bias at any level of correlation increases as the SD_r becomes larger relative to the SD_i.

Figure D-11 shows the effect of increasing the correlation between intakes and requirements, and at the same time changing the relative size of the SD_r when the EAR is equal to 70. In these cases, the true prevalence of inadequacy in the population is higher, as the EAR is now closer to the mean intake. Again, increasing SD_r appears to have a stronger effect on the bias of the prevalence estimator than does increasing the correlation between intakes and requirements.

Finally, Figure D-12 shows that when true prevalence is equal to 50 percent, neither increasing the correlation between intake and requirement nor increasing the relative size of SD_r has any effect on the bias of the prevalence estimate. The EAR cut-point method produces a correct prevalence estimate at any correlation level and for any value of the SD_r relative to the SD_i.

In summary, violating the independence assumption (i.e., a non-zero correlation) is likely to produce relatively minor biases on the estimates of prevalence obtained from applying the EAR cut-point method as long as the correlation between intakes and requirements does not exceed 0.5 or 0.6; the SD_r is substantially smaller than the SD_i; and the true prevalence is neither very small nor very large. The use of the EAR cut-point method (or the probability approach) is not recommended for investigating the adequacy of energy intakes in any group because for food energy the correlation between intakes and requirements is known to be very high.

VARIANCE OF REQUIREMENTS IS LARGE RELATIVE TO VARIANCE OF INTAKES

To test the effect of violating the assumption that variance of requirements must be substantially smaller than variance of intakes for good performance of the Estimated Average Requirement (EAR) cut-point method, various scenarios were considered. Mean intake was fixed at 90 units and SD_i at 30 units, as before, and 0.01 and 0.7 were chosen for the correlation between intakes and requirements. The EAR was fixed at three different values: 55, 70, and 90 units. For each of the six different scenarios, the SD_r varied from a low value of 0 to a high value of 40 units, in 5 unit increments.

Again, for each case, a large population was generated, and groups of 2,000 individuals were sampled 200 times. The prevalence estimates shown in each case are obtained as the average over the 200 replicates.

Box D-2 *Major findings—Variance of requirement relative to variance of intake*

• The impact of increasing the SD_r relative to the SD_i on the bias of the prevalence estimates can be large, especially when true prevalence is not close to 50 percent (Figures D-13 and D-15).

• When the correlation between intake and requirement is high (0.7), the bias in the estimated prevalence can be high, but it does not increase monotonically as SD_r increases (Figures D-14 and D-16).

• When true prevalence is 50 percent, increasing the SD_r even to values above the SD_i has no impact on the estimates of prevalence.

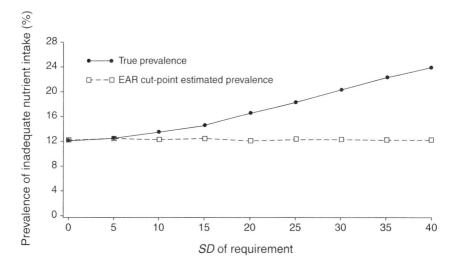

FIGURE D-13 Effect of the standard deviation of requirement (SD_r) on the estimated prevalence of inadequate intakes using the Estimated Average Requirement (EAR) cut-point method for 10 values of the SD_r. For all values of the SD_r, mean intake = 90, SD of intake = 30, EAR = 55, and correlation between intake and requirement = 0.01.

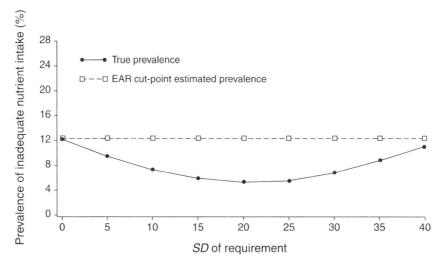

FIGURE D-14 Effect of the standard deviation of requirement (SD_r) on the estimated prevalence of inadequate intakes using the Estimated Average Requirement (EAR) cut-point method for 10 values of the SD_r. For all values of the SD_r, mean intake = 90, SD of intake = 30, EAR = 55, and correlation between intake and requirement = 0.7.

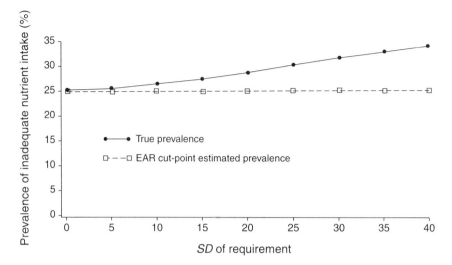

FIGURE D-15 Effect of the standard deviation of requirement (SD_r) on the estimated prevalence of inadequate intakes using the Estimated Average Requirement (EAR) cut-point method for 10 values of the SD_r. For all values of the SD_r, mean intake = 90, SD of intake = 30, EAR = 70, and correlation between intake and requirement = 0.01.

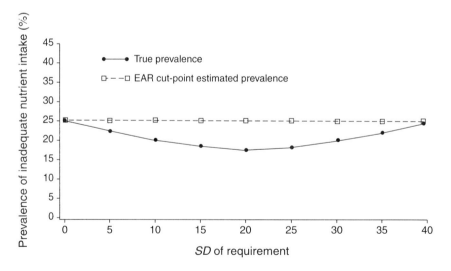

FIGURE D-16 Effect of the standard deviation of requirement (SD_r) on the estimated prevalence of inadequate intakes using the Estimated Average Requirement (EAR) cut-point method for 10 values of the SD_r. For all values of the SD_r, mean intake = 90, SD of intake = 30, EAR = 70, and correlation between intake and requirement = 0.7.

Figures D-17 and D-18 summarize the information presented in Figures D-13 through D-16. In Figure D-17, the three curves represent the bias of the prevalence estimate relative to the true prevalence for three values of the EAR and when the correlation between intakes and requirements is close to 0. The solid line with dots shows the expected bias when the EAR is 55 units for varying values of the SD_r. The dotted line with stars corresponds to the bias at varying values of SD_r when the EAR is 70. Finally, the dashed line with squares indicates the expected bias when the EAR is equal to the mean intake and the true prevalence is 50 percent. Notice that when SD_r is high relative to SD_i, the bias in the estimated prevalence can be substantial. Consider for example, the case where the EAR is 55 and the SD_r is 40. The bias in the estimated prevalence is approximately 11 percent. This might not seem significant until one recalls that for an SD_r of 30 and an EAR of 55, the true prevalence in the group is approximately 20 percent (see Figure D-1). Thus, the bias in the estimate of prevalence corresponds to a full 50 percent of the true prevalence in the population.

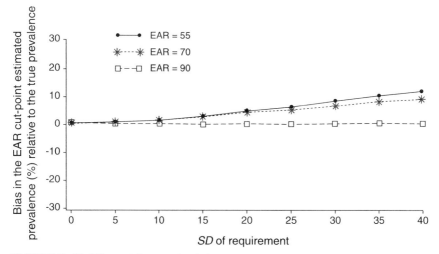

FIGURE D-17 Effect of the standard deviation of requirement (SD_r) on bias of the estimated prevalence of inadequate intakes using the Estimated Average Requirement (EAR) cut-point method for 10 values of the SD_r. For all values of the SD_r, mean intake = 90, SD of intake = 30, and correlation between intake and requirement = 0.01. The EAR was set at 55 units (solid line with dots), 70 units (dotted line with stars) and 90 units (dashed line with squares).

In Figure D-18, again the three curves represent the three different values of the EAR, but now the correlation between intakes and
requirements was fixed at 0.7. Referring back to Figures D-14 and
D-16, one can see that as the value of SD_r increases, the true prevalence first decreases and then increases. This is a result of the pattern of overlapping the requirements and intake distributions. The
biases in the estimates of prevalence shown in Figure D-18 follow
the same pattern. It is important to notice that the EAR cut-point
estimate of prevalence does not track the changes in true prevalence as the SD_r varies, and thus produces biased estimates.

In summary, violating the assumption requiring that the variance
of requirements be smaller than the variance of intakes is likely to
have a noticeable impact on the reliability of the prevalence estimate. To date, suggested estimates of the variance of requirements
for most nutrients are smaller than those calculated for intakes. In
principle, therefore, one need not worry about potential violations
of this assumption. A situation in which the variance of intake may
become small relative to the variance of requirements is for institu-

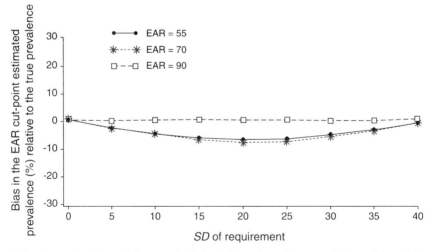

FIGURE D-18 Effect of the standard deviation of requirement (SD_r) on bias of the
estimated prevalence of inadequate intakes using the Estimated Average Requirement (EAR) cut-point method for 10 values of the SD_r. For all values of the SD_r,
mean intake = 90, SD of intake = 30, and correlation between intake and requirement = 0.7. The EAR was set at 55 units (solid line with dots), 70 units (dotted line
with stars) and 90 units (dashed line with squares).

tionalized populations, in which feeding is controlled and about the same for all individuals in the group (e.g., nursing homes). In these special instances it may be possible that the variance of intakes in the group could become small enough to create a problem. In this case, it might be better to assess adequacy using the probability approach rather than its short cut.

THE DISTRIBUTION OF REQUIREMENTS IS NOT SYMMETRICAL AROUND THE EAR

The assumption of symmetry of the requirement distribution is inappropriate for at least one important nutrient: iron requirements in menstruating women. As will be evident by inspection of the simulation results, when this assumption does not hold the performance of the Estimated Average Requirement (EAR) cut-point method for estimating the prevalence of nutrient inadequacy leaves much to be desired. In cases where it is known that the distribution of requirements is skewed, use of the probability approach is recommended to assess adequacy of nutrient intake for the group. In the case of iron, for example, the estimate of prevalence that would result from applying the probability approach and using a log-normal model for the requirement distribution will be less biased than that resulting from application of the EAR cut-point method. This is likely to be true even if the log-normal model is not the correct model for requirements.

The model used for simulating intakes and requirements in this section differs from the ones described in previous sections. Here, the simulation model was based on one proposed by the Food and Agriculture Organization/World Health Organization (FAO/WHO, 1988) to describe iron requirements. It has been established that daily losses of iron are 0.77 mg, and menstrual losses of iron are modeled as log-normal random variables with a mean (in natural log units) of –0.734 and standard deviation of 0.777. The specification of the model also assumes high iron availability in the diet (a bioavailability of 15 percent). For the simulation, the skewness of the requirement distribution was varied, and five values considered: 0.6, 1.3, 2.5, 3.2, and 5.7. Recall that for a symmetrical distribution, the value of the skewness coefficient is equal to zero; thus, increasing skewness reflects increasing departures from symmetry. Intakes were simulated independently as normal random variables with a mean intake of 12 mg, and standard deviation of 3 mg resulting in a CV of intake of 25 percent.

Rather than repeatedly sampling groups of 2,000 from the popu-

Box D-3   *Major findings—Distribution of requirements not symmetrical*

• The bias in the estimate of inadequacy that results from application of the EAR cut-point method when the distribution of requirements is skewed can be severe.
   • When skewness exceeds values around 2, the relative bias (estimated prevalence/true prevalence) is very large—over 100 percent.
   • Even though this simulation was limited in scope, results are striking enough for the Uses Subcommittee to recommend that the EAR cut-point method not be used to assess the prevalence of nutrient inadequacy for a nutrient with a skewed requirement distribution.

lation of 50,000, prevalence of inadequacy was estimated from the population itself. Therefore, the values shown in Table D-1 and in Figure D-19 represent the actual proportion of individuals with intakes below requirements (true prevalence) and the estimate obtained from application of the EAR cut-point method.

The only nutrient for which there is strong evidence indicating a skewed requirement distribution (at the time this report was published) is iron in menstruating women (FAO/WHO, 1988). In recent Institute of Medicine reports on Dietary Reference Intakes (DRIs)

TABLE D-1 True Prevalence of Inadequacy and Estimated Prevalence of Inadequacy of Iron Obtained Using the EAR Cut-point Method

Distribution of Requirements					
Mean	Standard Deviation	Skewness	True Prevalence (%)	Estimated Prevalence (%)	Bias(%)
8.4	0.7	0.62	12	11	1
8.6	1.4	1.32	15	11	4
9.0	2.5	2.51	20	11	9
9.5	3.9	3.15	24	11	13
10.4	6.9	5.73	28	12	16

NOTE: The distribution of usual intakes is fixed to be normal with a mean of 12 mg and a standard deviation of 3 mg.

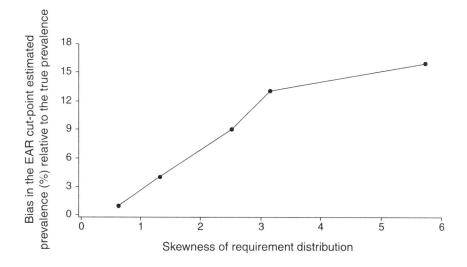

FIGURE D-19 The effect of the skewness of the requirement distribution on bias of the estimated prevalence of inadequate intakes using the Estimated Average Requirement (EAR) cut-point method for five values of skewness. For all levels of skewness, mean intake = 12 mg, standard deviation (*SD*) of intake = 3 mg, and correlation between intake and requirement = 0. The *SD* of requirement varied with the skewness of the requirement distribution.

no information was available to indicate nonsymmetrical distributions of requirements, so symmetry was assumed for the nutrients studied (IOM, 1997, 1998b, 2000).

   When requirements are not symmetrically distributed around the EAR, the probability approach should be used to assess prevalence of inadequacy. To implement the probability approach it is necessary to specify a probability model for the requirement distribution. The probability approach should result in essentially unbiased estimates of prevalence if a skewed requirement distribution is accurately specified. If the requirement distribution is incorrectly specified (for example, a log-normal model is chosen for estimation, but gamma or Weibull would be more correct), then the prevalence estimates obtained via the probability approach will also be biased. The effect of incorrect model specification on the bias of the probability approach has not been studied, but the bias resulting in this case would likely still be smaller than that resulting from the application of the EAR cut-point method to estimate prevalence.

E

Units of Observation: Assessing Nutrient Adequacy Using Household and Population Data

Typically, the unit of observation implicitly assumed in dietary assessment is the individual. That is, the analysis assumes that information is available on the usual intake of individuals. For either the probability approach or Estimated Average Requirement (EAR) cut-point method, data on individual intakes are compared with information on the distribution of individual requirements to estimate the prevalence of inadequacy in a group of individuals.

HOUSEHOLD-LEVEL ASSESSMENTS

In assessing the nutrient adequacy of household intakes, it is first necessary to construct a household requirement. It is important at this stage to be explicit about the intended application. One possibility is to evaluate the likely adequacy of intake for a specific household described in terms of the characteristics of each individual living in that household.

Energy

Using energy as an example, an estimate of the total energy need as a summation of the needs of the individuals in the household could be developed. In fact, the energy needs of particular individuals are not known, only the average of needs of similar individuals. By analogy the total need computed for the household from the Dietary Reference Intakes (DRIs) for individuals will have an associated variability. A joint 1985 report by the Food and Agriculture

232

Organization of the United Nations, World Health Organization, and United Nations University (FAO/WHO/UNU, 1985) on energy and protein requirements discussed the procedure for estimating the variance that should be attached to the household energy requirement estimate. In theory, a probability statement can be made about the likelihood of adequacy of the household energy intake. However, because of the expected correlation between energy intake and energy need, it will be difficult or impossible to interpret the probability unless the observed household intake falls well above or well below the distribution of needs of similar households. When this occurs there are serious limitations to the assessment of the estimated energy intake of a particular household and attempts to do so (with currently available methodology) are not recommended.

When the intended application is to assess the apparent adequacy of a population of households (e.g., in the examination of data from a household food use survey involving a large number of households), one can estimate the mean household energy requirement as a demographically weighted average—the summation of requirements for the typical household. In comparison with the description above, the variance of requirement would be increased to allow for the variation in household composition. A major distinction between assessing a particular household and assessing a population of households is that the population average household intake should be expected to approximate the population mean household energy requirement, thus the confidence associated with an assessment of the total group should be improved. Conversely, because of expected correlation between energy intakes and energy needs at the household level, it is not possible to generate an unbiased estimate of the prevalence of inadequate intakes. The issues are the same as those for assessment of populations of individuals.

Nutrients

Assessing the adequacy of intakes of other nutrients at the household level is also possible but the process is more complicated than for energy. Unlike for energy, where an aggregate household requirement can be generated, an aggregate household requirement cannot be used as an EAR for other nutrients because intake and requirement are not correlated for most nutrients. Even if household intake appears to meet the aggregate household need for the nutrient, the lack of correlation between intake and need suggests that there is no assurance that nutrient intakes will be distributed within the household in a manner likely to satisfy the needs of the individual household members.

This problem has been identified since at least 1970 when a Food and Agriculture Organization/World Health Organization (FAO/WHO) report on requirements of iron demonstrated that simply computing the aggregate requirement of household members did not begin to address issues of estimating the amount of iron that needed to be supplied *at the household level* if adequacy of intake of the individual family members was to be expected. That is, when a diet providing the aggregate iron need is acquired and consumed by the household, it is likely that food (and iron) will be distributed in proportion to energy needs of the individuals. As a result, there will almost certainly be serious shortfalls in iron intake for women and very young children and surplus iron intakes for adult men and boys (FAO/WHO, 1970). Although the problem had been identified, practical approaches to resolution were much later in coming.

A possible solution to this problem—suggested but not developed in the 1970 report—is to estimate the required nutrient density of the household diet such that when that diet is shared in proportion to energy, there is high likelihood that the needs of all individuals would be met. By definition, such a diet provided in amounts to meet household energy needs would represent a nutritionally adequate household-level diet. The required household nutrient density is set with respect to the class of individuals with the highest nutrient density need. With the use of current FAO/WHO nutrient and energy requirement estimates and the exclusion of pregnant women from the consideration, it turns out that this is often pubescent boys and girls or women of childbearing age.

The calculation of required nutrient density is not as simple as computing the ratio of either the Estimated Average Requirement (EAR) or Recommended Dietary Allowance (RDA) for the nutrient to the average energy requirement. The calculations must take into account variability of the nutrient requirement, expected variability of the nutrient density in ingested diets, and assurance of adequacy for the targeted individual. The theoretical basis for such calculations was partially developed by the 1985 FAO/WHO/UNU committee and an operational approach was subsequently applied by Beaton. In an unpublished report to the Canadian International Development Agency in 1995, Beaton operationalized these concepts in developing guidelines for fortification of foods for refugees where the household was taken as the unit of observation (and of distribution). Because household-level calculations are most likely to be conducted in connection with planning rather than evaluation, the technical aspect of the approach will be presented in a later report when planning is discussed.

With a reference nutrient density in hand, the proportion of households that meet two conditions can be calculated: an energy intake above the household level requirement and nutrient density above the reference. From this, as for assessment of groups of individuals, a prevalence of households with inadequate nutrient supplies and intakes may be computed. Note that the nutrient assessment can be meaningful only if household energy intake approximates the household energy need. This approach does not give an independent estimate of nutrient adequacy because if energy intake is inadequate for the total household, there can be no assurance that food (and nutrient intake) will be distributed in proportion to the energy needs of different classes of individuals—a core necessity of the nutrient density approach.

Although this approach can resolve some of the major issues when dealing with populations of households, it has severe limitations and is not recommended for assessment of observed intake of specific households.

A Caveat on Dietary Data Used for Household-Level Assessments

Although it is not within the purview of this report to address methodologies of food intake data collection, it is germane to warn about special issues to be considered in assessing the suitability of data or in developing adjustments. Information on household food consumption often comes from food *use* data, not from food *intake* data. Household food use refers to food and beverages used from household food purchases and supplies (stored foods, home production, etc.). Food use defined this way is not equivalent to food intake by individuals in the household. Food intake refers to foods actually eaten and is, in general, substantially less than food used by the household. Usage data must be adjusted (methods have been developed by the U.S. Department of Agriculture and others) to take into account food that is discarded and nutrient losses that may occur during storage, processing, and preparation (assuming that nutrient composition data relevant to foods as purchased rather than as consumed are used to compute energy and nutrient supply). Again the overriding principle is that both intakes and requirements must be expressed at the same level of aggregation and food preparation before valid comparisons can be made. Further, account must be taken of consumption of foods outside the household and whether these are included in the estimate of food use at the household level. If they are not included, the reference requirement figures may need to be changed.

POPULATION-LEVEL ASSESSMENTS

At the population level the most common method for assessing nutrient adequacy is based on food disappearance data (food balance sheets) (Gibson, 1990). For this discussion, all reservations are admitted but set aside about the validity of per capita energy and nutrient supplies calculated from food disappearance data and the allowances that are made for food wastage down to the retail level as well as wastage in the household. The Food and Agriculture Organization (FAO) and many national governments have devoted much effort to improving these procedures. Because the data serve many important purposes in the examination of food trade trends and supplies, computation of apparent nutrient supplies is a secondary or tertiary use of data.

Customary food balance sheets provide information on a country's food supply available for consumption derived from calculations based on estimates of amounts of domestic food produced plus food imports and any change in food stocks since the previous reference period, and less food exports and food diverted to non-human sectors (e.g., animal feeds) or converted to other forms in processing (e.g., alcohol production or in North America the production of high fructose sweeteners). Losses that must be taken into account include losses in the field, storage and transportation, and processing (taking into account any by-products that reenter the human food supply) and losses and wastage at the retail and household levels (garbage). Losses at the retail and household level vary widely between populations and perhaps population subgroups. Once the supply of food available for consumption is calculated, it is often converted to a per capita basis by dividing it by estimates of population size, although for energy assessment it might be expressed as the aggregate total energy supply (the units for intake and requirement must be the same for assessment purposes).

Uses of food balance sheets include the analysis of trends in a population's food supply, formulating changes in agricultural policies, and monitoring changes over time in the types of foods consumed (FAO, 1998). An additional reported use, perhaps implicit in the foregoing material, is using food balance sheet data to assess overall adequacy of the food supply relative to a population's nutritional requirements.

Per Capita Energy Needs

Historically, the goal has been to assess the apparent adequacy of total energy supply for a population or group of populations. An approach to the estimation of population energy needs was described in detail by James and Schofield (1990). Energy needs of each physiological stratum of the population—taking into account either actual or desirable body size and physical activity—are multiplied by the number of individuals in that stratum and these needs are aggregated for the population. Under the condition of overall adequacy judged against this estimate of aggregate need (which could be expressed as the total or per capita energy need), the assumption must be that, on a chronic basis, energy intake is distributed across strata and individuals in proportion to energy needs. If per capita supply meets or exceeds the per capita requirement (including allowance for wastage), then a satisfactory situation *can and should* exist. However, where total supply appears to fall short of total need, it must be accepted that the distribution of intakes is likely to be inequitable. Without information about that distribution, inferences cannot be drawn about the likely prevalence of inadequate intakes within the population. Interpretation is limited to the unit of observation—the population as a whole or sometimes a specific population subgroup for which food use data are available.

Per Capita Needs for Other Nutrients

In theory, one could also assess per capita intake data for adequacy of other nutrients at the population level. The approach would have to involve a first step of generating a per capita requirement probably based on an intermediate nutrient density approach as discussed above for household intake data. It is not certain whether such an approach has ever been attempted. Approaches based on a per capita recommended intake (e.g., demographically weighted Recommended Dietary Allowances [RDAs]) will *not* work for the same reasons discussed for household-level intake data. That is, it is unreasonable to assume equitable (proportional to actual need) distribution of nutrients. Methodologies for population-level assessment of nutrient supply are in their infancy and any attempt at such assessment should be scrutinized with great care. In the past the most commonly used approach was the simple comparison of per capita supply with the RDA, with or without even demographic weighting. That is an inappropriate use of the RDAs, past or present (Beaton, 1999).

In theory, then, an assessment of nutrient supply can be made with the population as the unit of observation but it would require very careful thought in building an estimate of the appropriate reference population requirement.

F

Rationale for Setting Adequate Intakes

In the Dietary Reference Intake (DRI) nutrient reports, the Adequate Intake (AI) has been estimated in a number of different ways. Because of this, the exact meanings and interpretations of the AIs differ. Some AIs have been based on the observed mean intake of groups or subpopulations that are maintaining health and nutritional status consistent with meeting the criteria for adequacy. However, where reliable information about these intakes was not available, or where there were conflicting data, other approaches were used. As a result, the definition of an AI is broad and includes experimentally estimated desirable intakes.

These varying methods of setting an AI make using the AI for assessing intakes of groups difficult. When the AI is based directly on intakes of apparently healthy populations, it is correct to assume that other populations (with similar distributions of intakes) have a low prevalence of inadequate intakes if the mean intake is at or above the AI. For nutrients for which the AI was not based on intakes of apparently healthy populations, a group mean intake at or above the AI would still indicate a low prevalence of inadequate intakes for that group but there is less confidence in this assessment. Tables F-1 through F-6 give more details on the methods used to set the AIs for calcium, vitamin D, fluoride, pantothenic acid, biotin, and choline. For infants, AIs have been set for all nutrients evaluated to date (see table at the end of this book). For all these nutrients except vitamin D, the AI for infants is based on intakes of healthy populations that are fed only human milk. How-

239

ever, for the other age groups, only fluoride and pantothenic acid AIs are based on intakes of apparently healthy populations.

TABLE F-1 Adequate Intake (AI) for Calcium

Life Stage Group	AI (mg/d)	Basis for AI
0–6 mo	210	Human milk content
7–12 mo	270	Human milk content + solid food
1–3 y	500	Extrapolation from AI for 4–8 y (desirable calcium retention)
4–8 y	800	Calcium balance, calcium accretion, ΔBMC[b]
9–18 y	1,300	Desirable calcium retention, ΔBMC, factorial
19–30 y	1,000	Desirable calcium retention, factorial
31–50 y	1,000	Calcium balance, BMD[c]

Study Population[a]

Balance studies:

n=60 girls and 39 boys; aged 2–8 y; normal and healthy (Matkovic, 1991; Matkovic and Heaney, 1992)

Retention studies:

1. n=115 girls and 113 boys; aged 9–19 y (Martin et al., 1997)
2. n=80; aged 12–15 y; Caucasians (Greger et al., 1978; Jackman et al., 1997; Matkovic et al., 1990)
3. n=111 girls and 22 boys; aged 9–17 y; normal and healthy (Matkovic and Heaney, 1992)

BMC studies:

1. n=94 Caucasian girls; mean age 12 y (Lloyd et al., 1993)
2. n=48 Caucasian girls; mean age 11 y (Chan et al., 1995)
3. n=70 pairs of identical twins; aged 6–14 y; 45 pairs completed the 3-y study (Johnston et al., 1992)

n=26 men and 137 women; aged 18–30 y; normal and healthy (Matkovic and Heaney, 1992)

Balance studies:

1. n=130 premenopausal women (white Roman Catholic nuns); aged 35–50 y (Heaney et al., 1977)
2. n=25 healthy women; aged 30–39 y (Ohlson et al., 1952)
3. n=34 healthy women; aged 40–49 y (Ohlson et al., 1952)

BMD studies:

1. n=37 premenopausal women; aged 30–42 y (Baran et al., 1990)
2. n=49 premenopausal, healthy women; aged 46–55 y; Netherlands (Elders et al., 1994)

continued

TABLE F-1 Adequate Intake (AI) for Calcium

Life Stage Group	AI (mg/d)	Basis for AI
51–70 y	1,200	Desirable calcium retention, factorial, ΔBMD
> 70 y	1,200	Extrapolation from AI for 51–70 y (desirable calcium retention), ΔBMD, fracture rate
Pregnancy and lactation, <18 y	1,300	Bone mineral mass
Pregnancy and lactation, 19–50 y	1,000	Bone mineral mass

[a] Unless noted otherwise, all studies were performed in the United States or Canada.
[b] ΔBMC = change in bone mineral content.
[c] ΔBMD = change in bone mineral density.

Study Population[a]

Retention studies:

1. $n=85$ women with vertebral osteoporosis; aged 48–77 y (Hasling et al., 1990)
2. $n=18$ women and 7 men with osteoporosis; aged 26–70 y, mean age 53 (Selby, 1994)
3. $n=181$ balance studies of ambulatory men; aged 34–71 y, mean age 54 (Spencer et al., 1984)
4. $n=76$ women; aged 50–85 y (Ohlson et al., 1952)
5. $n=61$ postmenopausal women with osteoporosis (Marshall et al., 1976)
6. $n=41$ postmenopausal, estrogen-deprived women (white Roman Catholic nuns); mean age 46 y (Heaney and Recker, 1982; Heaney et al., 1978)

BMD studies:

1. $n=9$ clinical trials in postmenopausal women (Aloia et al., 1994; Chevalley et al., 1994; Dawson-Hughes et al., 1990; Elders et al., 1991; Prince et al., 1991, 1995; Recker et al., 1996; Reid et al., 1995; Riis et al., 1987)
2. $n=77$ men; aged 30–87 y, mean age 58; 3-y study (Orwoll et al., 1990)

TABLE F-2 Adequate Intake (AI) for Vitamin D

Life Stage Group	AI (µg/d)	Basis for AI
0–6 mo	5	Serum 25(OH)D[b] level
7–12 mo	5	Serum 25(OH)D level
1–3 y 4–8 y 9–13 y 14–18 y	5	Serum 25(OH)D level
19–50 y	5	Serum 25(OH)D level
51–70 y	10	Serum 25(OH)D level
>70 y	15	Serum 25(OH)D level
Pregnancy and lactation, all ages	5	Serum 25(OH)D level

[a] Unless noted otherwise, all studies were performed in the United States or Canada.
[b] 25(OH)D = 25-hydroxyvitamin D.

Study Population[a]

$n=$ 256 full-term Chinese infants (Specker et al., 1992)

1. $n=18$ healthy, full-term, human-milk-fed infants; 17 Caucasian, 1 Asian-Indian (Greer et al., 1982)
2. $n=150$ normal, full-term, formula-fed Chinese infants (Leung et al., 1989)
3. $n=38$ healthy infants, aged 6–12 months; Norway (Markestad and Elzouki, 1991)

1. $n=104$ boys and 87 girls; healthy, normal; aged 8–18 y; Norway (Aksnes and Aarskog, 1982)
2. $n=90$ randomly selected school students in Turkey; 41 girls, 49 boys; aged 6–17 y (Gultekin et al., 1987)

1. $n=52$ women; aged 25–35 y (Kinyamu et al., 1997)

1. $n=247$ healthy, postmenopausal, ambulatory women; mean age 64 y (Dawson-Hughes et al., 1995)
2. $n=333$ healthy, postmenopausal, Caucasian women; mean age 58 y (Krall et al., 1989)
3. $n=249$ healthy, postmenopausal, ambulatory women; mean age 62 y (Dawson-Hughes et al., 1991)

1. $n=60$ women living in a nursing home, mean age 84 y; and 64 free-living women, mean age 71 y (Kinyamu et al., 1997)
2. $n=109$ men and women living in a nursing home; mean age 82 y (O'Dowd et al., 1993)
3. $n=116$ men and women; mean age 81 y (Gloth et al., 1995)

TABLE F-3 Adequate Intake (AI) for Fluoride

Life Stage Group	AI (mg/d)[a]	Basis for AI
0–6 mo	0.01	Human milk content
7–12 mo	0.5	Caries prevention
1–3 y	0.7	Caries prevention
4–8 y	1	Caries prevention
9–13 y	2	Caries prevention
14–18 y, males	3	Caries prevention
14–18 y, females	3	Caries prevention
>19 y, males	4	Caries prevention
>19 y, females	3	Caries prevention
Pregnancy and lactation, <18 y	3	Caries prevention
Pregnancy and lactation, 19–50 y	3	Caries prevention

[a] For all life stage groups, the AI was calculated using 0.05 mg/kg/day as the amount of fluoride needed to prevent dental caries. This amount was based on the studies outlined in this table.
[b] Unless noted otherwise, all studies were performed in the United States or Canada.

Study Population[b]

Caries prevention was based on the following studies that measured or
calculated fluoride intake in children:
1. number of infants not given; aged 1–9 y (McClure, 1943)
2. calculated total daily fluoride intake for a typical infant at age 2, 4, and 6
   mo using food analyses and caloric intake estimates (Singer and Ophaug,
   1979)
3. calculated average daily fluoride intake for a typical 6-mo-old infant and 2-y-
   old child using U.S. Food and Drug Administration food consumption
   estimates and food analyses; calculations were done for four dietary regions
   in the United States (Ophaug et al., 1980a, b, 1985)
4. calculated fluoride intake from 24-h dietary recalls of 250 mothers as part of
   Nutrition Canada Survey (Dabeka et al., 1982)

Caries prevention was based on the following studies which measured or
calculated fluoride intake in adults:
1. analyzed duplicate diets of 24 adults and determined mean dietary intake
   (Dabeka et al., 1987)
2. analyzed hospital diet; $n=93$ food items (Taves, 1983)
3. measured dietary intake of 10 adult male hospital patients (Spencer et al.,
   1981)
4. calculated total daily intake for typical males aged 15–19 y using food
   composition and consumption data (Singer et al., 1980, 1985)
5. determined average daily intake from analysis of hospital diet; $n=287$ diets
   (Osis et al., 1974)
6. calculated daily intake from food analyses of diets from 16 U.S. cities
   (Kramer et al., 1974)

TABLE F-4 Adequate Intake (AI) for Pantothenic Acid

Life Stage Group	AI (mg/d)	Basis for AI
0–6 mo	1.7	Human milk content
7–12 mo	1.8	Mean of extrapolation from AI for 0–6 mo and adult AI[b]
1–3 y	2	Extrapolation from adult AI
4–8 y	3	Extrapolation from adult AI
9–13 y	4	Extrapolation from adult AI
14–18 y	5	Extrapolation from adult AI, urinary pantothenate excretion
≥ 19 y	5	Usual intake
Pregnancy, all ages	6	Usual intake
Lactation, all ages	7	Usual intake, maternal blood concentrations, secretion of pantothenic acid into milk

[a] Unless noted otherwise, all studies were performed in the United States or Canada.
[b] To extrapolate from the AI for adults to an AI for children, the following formula is used $AI_{child} = AI_{adult}$ (F), where F = (Weight$_{child}$/Weight$_{adult}$)$^{0.75}$ (1 + growth factor). To extrapolate from the AI for infants ages 0–6 months to an AI for infants ages 7–12 months, the following formula is used: $AI_{7-12\ mo} = AI_{0-6\ mo}$ (F), where F = (Weight$_{7-12\ mo}$/Weight$_{0-6\ mo}$)$^{0.75}$.

Study Population[a]

1. n=26 boys aged 14–19 y and 37 girls aged 13–17 y; all healthy volunteers (Eissenstat et al., 1986)
2. n=8 boys and 4 girls; aged 11–16 y (Kathman and Kies, 1984)

Usual intake was based on 4 studies:
1. n=23 (16 females, 7 males), aged 18–53 y (mean 26 y), 19 Caucasian, 4 Chinese, all normal healthy volunteers (Kathman and Kies, 1984)
2. n=7,277 randomly selected British households from the U.K. National Food Survey (Bull and Buss, 1982)
3. n=37 males, 54 females (26 institutionalized, 65 noninstitutionalized), aged 65+ y (Srinivasan et al., 1981)
4. n=12 healthy men, half were aged 21–35 y and half were aged 65–79 y (Tarr et al., 1981)

TABLE F-5 Adequate Intake (AI) for Biotin

Life Stage Group	AI (μg/d)	Basis for AI
0–6 mo	5	Human milk content
7–12 mo	6	Extrapolation from AI for 0–6 mo[a]
1–3 y	8	Extrapolation from AI for 0–6 mo[b]
4–8 y	12	Extrapolation from AI for 0–6 mo[b]
9–13 y	20	Extrapolation from AI for 0–6 mo[b]
14–18 y	25	Extrapolation from AI for 0–6 mo[b]
Adults, all ages	30	Extrapolation from AI for 0–6 mo[c]
Pregnancy, all ages	30	Extrapolation from AI for 0–6 mo
Lactation, all ages	35	Extrapolation from AI for 0–6 mo + amount of biotin secreted into milk

[a] To extrapolate from the AI for infants ages 0–6 months to an AI for infants ages 7–12 months, the following formula is used: $AI_{7-12\ mo} = AI_{0-6\ mo}\ (F)$, where $F = (Weight_{7-12\ mo}/Weight_{0-6\ mo})^{0.75}$.

[b] To extrapolate from the AI for infants ages 0-6 months to an AI for children and adolescents 1-18 years, the following formula is used: $AI_{child} = AI_{0-6\ mo}\ (F)$, where $F = (Weight_{child}/Weight_{0-6\ mo})^{0.75}$.

[c] To extrapolate from the AI for infants ages 0-6 months to an AI for adults, the following formula is used: $AI_{adult} = AI_{0-6\ mo}\ (F)$, where $F = (Weight_{adult}/Weight_{0-6\ mo})^{0.75}$.

Study Population

1. $n= 35$ mature milk samples from 38 healthy nursing mothers in Japan (Hirano et al., 1992)
2. $n=140$ healthy, full-term infants in Finland; 4 mo lactation (Salmenpera et al., 1985)

TABLE F-6 Adequate Intake (AI) for Choline

Life Stage Group	AI (mg/d)	Basis for AI
0–6 mo	125	Human milk content
7–12 mo	150	Extrapolation from AI for 0–6 mo[a]
1–3 y	200	Extrapolation from adult AI
4–8 y	250	Extrapolation from adult AI
9–13 y	375	Extrapolation from adult AI
14–18 y, males	550	Extrapolation from adult AI
14–18 y, females	400	Extrapolation from adult AI
≥19 y, males	550	Prevention of ALT[b] abnormalities
≥19 y, females	425	Prevention of ALT abnormalities
Pregnancy, all ages	450	Prevention of ALT abnormalities + cost of pregnancy
Lactation, all ages	550	Prevention of ALT abnormalities + amount of choline secreted into milk

[a] To extrapolate from the AI for adults to an AI for children, the following formula is used $AI_{child} = AI_{adult}$ (F), where $F = (Weight_{child}/Weight_{adult})^{0.75}$ (1 + growth factor). To extrapolate from the AI for infants ages 0–6 months to an AI for infants ages 7–12 months, the following formula is used: $AI_{7-12\ mo} = AI_{0-6\ mo}$ (F), where $F = (Weight_{7-12\ mo}/Weight_{0-6\ mo})^{0.75}$.

[b] ALT = alanine aminotransferase.

Study Population

n=16 healthy male volunteers; aged 29 y (Zeisel et al., 1991)

G
Glossary and Abbreviations

Acute exposure

An exposure to a toxin or excess amount of a nutrient that is short term, perhaps as short as one day or one dose. In this report it generally refers to total exposure (diet plus supplements) on a single day.

Adequacy of nutrient intake

Intake of a nutrient that meets the individual's requirement for that nutrient.

Adverse effects

In the toxicological sense, defined symptoms of poor or undesirable health resulting from administration of a toxin or excess amounts of a nutrient.

AI

Adequate Intake; a recommended intake value based on observed or experimentally determined approximations or estimates of nutrient intake by a group (or groups) of apparently healthy people that are assumed to be adequate—used when an RDA cannot be determined.

Bias

Used in a statistical sense, referring to a tendency of an estimate to deviate from a true value (as by reason of nonrandom sampling). To be unbiased, a statistic would have an expected value equal to a population parameter being estimated.

Chronic exposure

Exposure to a chemical compound such as a nutrient for a long period of time, perhaps as long as every day for the lifetime of an individual.

Cluster analysis

A general approach to multivariate problems, the aim of which is to determine whether individuals fall into groups or clusters.

Cut-point

The exact point when something stops or changes. The EAR is used as a cut-point in the EAR cut-point method of assessing the prevalence of inadequacy for a group.

Deficiency

An abnormal physiological condition resulting from inadequate intake of a nutrient or multiple nutrients.

Dietary reference standards

Nutrient intake values established as goals for individuals or groups for good nutrition and health.

Dietary status

The condition of an individual or group as a result of food and nutrient intake. Dietary status also refers to the sum of dietary intake measurements for an individual or a group.

Disappearance data

Data that refer to food and nutrients that disappear from the marketplace. The term refers to food and nutrient availability for a population that is calculated from national or regional statistics by the inventory-style method. Usually taken into account are the sum of food remaining from the previous year, food imports, and agricultural production; from this sum is subtracted the sum of food remaining at the end of the year, food exports, food waste, and food used for non-food purposes. Disappearance data do not always take account of food that does not enter commerce, such as home food production, wild food harvests, etc.

Distribution of observed intakes	The observed dietary or nutrient intake distribution representing the variability of *observed* intakes in the population of interest. For example, the distribution of observed intakes may be obtained from dietary survey data such as 24-hour recalls.
Distribution of requirements	The distribution reflecting the individual-to-individual variability in requirements. Variability exists because not all individuals in a (sub)population have the same requirements for a nutrient (even if individuals are grouped into homogenous classes, such as Hispanic men aged 19 to 50 years).
Distribution of usual intakes	The distribution of long-run average dietary or nutrient intakes of individuals in the population. The distribution should reflect only the individual-to-individual variability in intakes. Statistical procedures may be used to adjust the distribution of observed intakes by partially removing the day-to-day variability in individual intakes, so the adjusted distribution more closely reflects a usual intake distribution.
Dose-response assessment	Determines the relationship between nutrient intake (dose) and either some criterion of adequacy or adverse effect.
DRI	Dietary Reference Intake; a reference value that is a quantitative estimate of a nutrient intake. It is used for planning and assessing diets for healthy people.
EAR	Estimated Average Requirement; a nutrient intake estimated to meet the requirement of half the healthy individuals in a particular life stage and gender group.

EAR cut-point method	A method of assessing the nutrient adequacy of groups. It consists of assessing the proportion of individuals in the group whose usual nutrient intakes are below the EAR.
Error in measurement	Mistake made in the observation or recording of data.
Food balance sheet	See disappearance data.
Former RDA and RNI	Recommended daily dietary intake level of a nutrient sufficient to meet the nutrient requirement of nearly all healthy persons in a particular life stage and gender group. These standards were last issued in the United States in 1989 (RDA, Recommended Dietary Allowance) and in Canada in 1990 (RNI, Recommended Nutrient Intake).
Household	Individuals sharing in the purchase, preparation, and consumption of foods. Usually this will represent individuals living as a family in one home, including adults and children. A household may be the unit of observation rather than the independent individuals within it.
Inadequacy of nutrient intake	Intake of a nutrient that fails to meet the individual's requirement for that nutrient.
Interindividual variability	Variability from person-to-person.
Intraindividual variability	Variability within one person. The term is generally used to refer to day-to-day variation in reported intakes, also called the within-person variation or standard deviation within (SD_{within}).
Joint distribution	Simultaneous distribution of both requirements (y-axis) and usual intakes (x-axis) for a single nutrient by individuals within a population or group.

Likelihood	Probability.
LOAEL	Lowest-observed-adverse-effect level; lowest intake (or experimental dose) of a nutrient at which an adverse effect has been identified.
Mean intake	Average intake of a particular nutrient or food for a group or population of individuals. Also average intake of a nutrient or food over two or more days for an individual.
Mean requirement	Average requirement of a particular nutrient for a group or population of individuals.
NOAEL	No-observed-adverse-effect level; the highest intake (or experimental dose) of a nutrient at which no adverse effects have been observed in the individuals studied.
Normal distribution	In the statistical sense, refers to a specific type of distribution of the values for a parameter within a group or population. The distribution is symmetrical and the mean ± 2 standard deviations will encompass the parameter for 95 percent of the individuals in the group.
Nutrient requirement	The lowest continuing intake level of a nutrient that will maintain a defined level of nutriture in a healthy individual; also called individual requirement.
Nutritional status	Condition of an individual or group resulting from nutrient intake and utilization of a nutrient at the tissue level.
Population	A large group; in this report, a large group of people.
Prevalence	The percentage of a defined population that is affected by a specific condition at the same time.

Prevalence of inadequate intakes	The percentage of a population that has intakes below requirements.
Probability approach	A method of assessing the nutrient adequacy of groups. It uses the distribution of usual intakes and the distribution of requirements to estimate the prevalence of inadequate intakes in a group. Also known as the NRC approach.
Probability of inadequacy	Outcome of a calculation that compares an individual's usual intake to the distribution of requirements for persons of the same life stage and gender to determine the probability that the individual's intake does not meet his or her requirement.
RDA	Recommended Dietary Allowance; the average daily intake level sufficient to meet the nutrient requirement of nearly all (97 to 98 percent) healthy individuals in a particular life stage and gender group.
Requirement	The lowest continuing intake level of a nutrient that will maintain a defined level of nurture in a healthy individual.
Risk	The probability or likelihood that some unwanted effect will occur; in this report, refers to an unwanted effect from too small or too large an intake of a nutrient.
Risk assessment	A scientific undertaking to characterize the nature and likelihood of harm resulting from human exposure to agents in the environment (in this case, a dietary nutrient). It includes both qualitative and quantitative information and a discussion of the scientific uncertainties in that information. The process of risk assessment can be divided into four major steps: hazard identification, dose-response assessment, exposure assessment, and risk characterization.

Risk curve	Used to demonstrate inadequacy or excess of a particular nutrient. As defined in the usual statistical sense, a risk curve is in contrast to the concept of probability curve.
Risk of excess	In relation to the DRIs, the likelihood that an individual will exceed the UL for a particular nutrient.
Risk of exposure	In the toxicological sense, the likelihood that individuals will experience contact with a toxin (or consume levels of a nutrient above the UL).
Risk of inadequacy	The likelihood that an individual will have usual intake of a particular nutrient that is less than the individual's requirement.
Sensitivity analysis	Technique of varying the implicit assumptions or presumed conditions of an analysis approach to see how much this affects the overall outcome.
Skewed distribution	A distribution that is not symmetrical around its mean. For example, a skewed distribution can have a long tail to the right (right-skewed distribution) or to the left (left-skewed distribution).
Symmetrical distribution	A distribution that has the same number of values (observations) above and below the mean and has equal proportions of these values around the mean.
Threshold	The point in a dose-response curve that is accepted as the point beyond which a risk of adverse effects occurs.
Toxicity	An adverse condition relating to or caused by a toxin.

True prevalence	The actual prevalence of a condition assuming no error in measurement of either requirements or intakes that would result in false negative or false positive classifications.
UF	Uncertainty factor; a value assigned to a specific nutrient reflecting the level of uncertainty about data used to establish a Tolerable Upper Intake Level.
UL	Tolerable Upper Intake Level; the highest average daily nutrient intake level likely to pose no risk of adverse health effects to almost all individuals in the general population. As intake increases above the UL, the potential risk of adverse effects increases.
Unit of observation	The level of aggregation at which data are collected. For example, the unit of observation for dietary assessment may be the individual, the household, or the population.
Univariate distribution	The distribution of a single variable.
Usual intake	The long-run average intake of food, nutrients, or a specific nutrient for an individual.
Variance of usual intakes or requirements	In the statistical sense, reflects the spread of the distribution of usual intakes or requirements on both sides of the mean intake or requirement. When the variance of a distribution is low, the likelihood of seeing values that are far away from the mean is low; in contrast, when the variance is large, the likelihood of seeing values that are far away from the mean is high. For usual intakes and requirements, variance reflects the person-to-person variability in the group.

H
Biographical Sketches of Subcommittee Members

SUZANNE P. MURPHY, Ph.D., R.D. (*Chair*), is a researcher at the Cancer Research Center of Hawaii at the University of Hawaii, Honolulu. Previously, she was an adjunct associate professor in the Department of Nutritional Sciences at the University of California at Berkeley and director of the California Expanded Food and Nutrition Program at the University of California at Davis. She received her B.S. in mathematics from Temple University and her Ph.D. in nutrition from the University of California at Berkeley. Dr. Murphy's research interests include dietary assessment methodology, development of food composition databases, and nutritional epidemiology. She was a member of the National Nutrition Monitoring Advisory Council and serves on the editorial boards of the *Journal of Nutrition, Journal of Food Composition and Analysis, Family Economics and Nutrition Review,* and *Nutrition Today.* Dr. Murphy is a member of numerous professional organizations including the American Dietetic Association, American Society for Nutritional Sciences, American Public Health Association, American Society for Clinical Nutrition, and Society for Nutrition Education. She has over 50 publications on dietary assessment methodology and has lectured nationally and internationally on this subject.

LENORE ARAB, Ph.D., is a professor of epidemiology and nutrition in the Departments of Epidemiology and Nutrition at the University of North Carolina at Chapel Hill School of Public Health. Dr. Arab's main research interests are anticarcinogens in foods, heterocyclic amines, breast cancer incidence and survival, the rela-

262

tionship of diet to atherosclerosis, antioxidant nutrients in various diseases, iron nutriture, and multimedia approaches to dietary assessment. She has published over 140 original papers as well as numerous book chapters and monographs. Dr. Arab serves as a nutrition advisor to the World Health Organization (WHO) and is the founding director of the WHO Collaborating Center for Nutritional Epidemiology in Berlin. She is the North American Editor of the journal *Public Health Nutrition* and sits on the editorial boards of the *European Journal of Clinical Nutrition, Journal of Clinical Epidemiology*, and *Public Health Nutrition*. Dr. Arab received her M.Sc. from the Harvard School of Public Health and her Ph.D. in nutrition from Justus Liebig University in Giessen, Germany.

SUSAN I. BARR, Ph.D., R.D., is a professor of nutrition at the University of British Columbia. She received a Ph.D. in human nutrition from the University of Minnesota and is a registered dietitian in Canada. Her research interests focus on the associations among nutrition, physical activity, and bone health in women, and she has authored over 60 publications. Dr. Barr has served as vice president of the Canadian Dietetic Association (now Dietitians of Canada) and is a fellow of both the Dietitians of Canada and the American College of Sports Medicine. She is currently a member of the Scientific Advisory Board of the Osteoporosis Society of Canada, the Medical Advisory Board of the Milk Processors Education Program, and the Scientific Advisory Board of Canada's National Institute of Nutrition.

SUSAN T. BORRA, R.D., is senior vice president and director of nutrition at the International Food Information Council. Ms. Borra is responsible for directing communications programs, executing public affairs strategies, and managing nutrition and food safety issues. Additionally, she oversees the development of consumer education materials and nutrition, food safety, and health programs. Ms. Borra is President-elect of the American Dietetic Association, past chair of the American Dietetic Association Foundation, and is a member of the American Heart Association and the Society for Nutrition Education. She has a bachelor's degree in nutrition and dietetics from the University of Maryland and is a registered dietitian.

ALICIA L. CARRIQUIRY, Ph.D., is an associate provost and associate professor in the Department of Statistics at Iowa State University. She has a Ph.D. in statistics and animal science from Iowa State. Since 1990, Dr. Carriquiry has been a consultant for the U.S.

Department of Agriculture Human Nutrition Information Service. She has also done consulting for the U.S. Environmental Protection Agency, the National Pork Producers Council, and is an affiliate for the Law and Economics Consulting Group. At present, Dr. Carriquiry is investigating the statistical issues associated with the Third National Health and Nutrition Examination Survey (NHANES III) and she has recently completed reports on improving the USDA's food intake surveys and methods to estimate adjusted intake, and biochemical measurement distributions for NHANES III. Dr. Carriquiry is the current Program Chair of the International Society for Bayesian Analysis and is an elected member of the International Statistical Institute. She is editor of *Statistical Science*, and serves on the Board of Directors of the National Institute of Statistical Science and of the International Society for Bayesian Analysis. Her research interests include nutrition and dietary assessment, Bayesian methods and applications, mixed models and variance component estimation.

BARBARA L. DEVANEY, Ph.D., is an economist and senior fellow at Mathematica Policy Research in Princeton, New Jersey. Her substantive expertise is in the areas of food assistance and nutrition policy and child health policy and programs. She has conducted several studies of the school nutrition programs, the Food Stamp Program, and the Special Supplemental Nutrition Program for Women, Infants and Children (WIC). Dr. Devaney also serves on the advisory board for the Maternal and Child Health Nutrition Leadership Training Program and was Visiting Professor for UCLA's program where she taught classes on food and nutrition assistance policy. She previously served as a member of the Institute of Medicine's Committee on Scientific Evaluation of the WIC Nutrition Risk Criteria. Dr. Devaney received her Ph.D. in economics from the University of Michigan.

JOHANNA T. DWYER, D.Sc., R.D., is director of the Frances Stern Nutrition Center at New England Medical Center and professor in the Departments of Medicine and of Community Health at the Tufts Medical School and School of Nutrition Science and Policy in Boston. She is also senior scientist at the Jean Mayer U.S. Department of Agriculture Human Nutrition Research Center on Aging at Tufts University. Dr. Dwyer's work centers on life cycle-related concerns such as the prevention of diet-related disease in children and adolescents and maximization of quality of life and health in elderly adults. She also has a long-standing interest in vegetarian and other alternative lifestyles. Dr. Dwyer is currently the editor of *Nutrition*

Today and on the editorial boards of *Family Economics and Nutrition Review* and *Nutrition Reviews*. She received her D.Sc. and M.Sc. from the Harvard School of Public Health, an M.S. from the University of Wisconsin, and her undergraduate degree with distinction from Cornell University. She is a member of the Institute of Medicine, the Food and Nutrition Board's Standing Committee on the Scientific Evaluation of Dietary Reference Intakes, past president of the American Society for Nutrition Sciences, past secretary of the American Society for Clinical Nutrition, and a past president of the Society for Nutrition Education.

JEAN-PIERRE HABICHT, M.D., Ph.D., is a professor of nutritional epidemiology in the Division of Nutrition Sciences at Cornell University. His professional experience includes serving as special assistant to the director of the Division of Health Examination Statistics at the National Center for Health Statistics, World Health Organization (WHO) medical officer at the Instituto de Nutricion de Centro America y Panama, and professor of maternal and child health at the University of San Carlos in Guatemala. Currently, Dr. Habicht serves as an advisor to United Nations (UN) and government health and nutrition agencies. He is a member of the WHO Expert Advisory Panel on Nutrition and the UN Advisory Group on Nutrition. He has consulted for the UN World Food Program and is involved in research with the UN High Commission for Refugees about the adequacy of food rations in refugee camps. Dr. Habicht served as a member of the Institute of Medicine's Food and Nutrition Board (1981–1984) and as a member and past chair of the Committee on International Nutrition Programs. Dr. Habicht chaired the National Research Council's Coordinating Committee on Evaluation of Food Consumption Surveys which produced the 1986 report, *Nutrient Adequacy: Assessment Using Food Consumption Surveys.*

HARRIET V. KUHNLEIN, Ph.D., R.D., is professor of human nutrition in the School of Dietetics and Human Nutrition at McGill University and Founding Director of the Centre for Indigenous Peoples' Nutrition and Environment. She is a registered dietitian in Canada and holds a Ph.D. in nutrition from the University of California at Berkeley. The focus of Dr. Kuhnlein's research is on the nutrition, food habits, and environment of indigenous peoples. Specifically, her work examines the traditional foods of indigenous peoples, contaminant levels in indigenous Arctic food systems, and nutrition promotion programs for indigenous peoples. She has published numerous articles on these subjects. Dr. Kuhnlein is a member of both the American and Canadian Societies of Nutritional Sciences, the Society for International Nutrition Research, the Canadian Dietetic Association, and the Society for Nutrition Education. She serves on the advisory council of the Herb Research Foundation and is a former cochair of the committee on Nutrition and Anthropology of the International Union of Nutritional Sciences. Dr. Kuhnlein also serves on the editorial boards of *Ecology of Food and Nutrition, Journal of Food Composition and Analysis, Journal of Ethnobiology,* and the *International Journal of Circumpolar Health.*

Index

A

Acute exposure, 254
Adequacy of nutrient intake
    confidence levels, 6, 56-57, 60, 64-65, 67, 68, 189-190, 197, 199, 200
    criteria of, 23, 27
    defined, 254
    household level, 233-234
    in individual-level assessments, 6, 56-57, 60, 64-65, 67, 68, 189-190, 197, 199, 200
    observed difference and, 187
    probability of correct conclusion about, 190, 199
    risk-reduction based indicator of, 2, 23, 27
    uncertainty in, 186, 188-189
Adequate Intakes (AIs). *See also specific nutrients*
    adaptations in, 26
    applicable population, 26
    context for use, 23, 24, 25, 111
    defined, 3, 106, 239, 254
    derivation of, 25, 26, 27, 106-109
    EARs compared, 59, 109, 163, 198
    extrapolation from other age groups, 26
    and food guides, 38
    in group-level assessments, 4, 12, 106, 109-112

    and group mean intake, 6, 12, 107, 108, 110, 111, 131
    indicators used to set, 27, 107-109
    in individual-level assessments, 4, 6-7, 46, 51, 58-62, 67, 68, 69, 194, 198-200
    limitations in dietary assessment, 4, 109-112
    methods used to set, 239-253
    misuse of, 111-112
    nutrients, by life-stage groups, 107-109, 240-253, 274-275
    and prevalence of inadequate intakes, 12, 109-110
    pseudo EAR calculated from, 111-112
    qualitative interpretation of intakes relative to, 62
    RDAs compared, 26-27, 59, 109, 198
    risk of inadequacy, 59
    uses, 25, 30
    usual intakes above or below, 46, 59-60, 110, 126
Adjusted standardized intakes, 137
Adjusting intake distributions
    day-to-day correlation in data and, 9, 96, 196-197
    heterogeneous within-person variation and, 95
    Iowa State University method, 98-102, 160

267

O

P

FOOD AND NUTRITION BOARD, INSTITUTE OF MEDICINE—
NATIONAL ACADEMY OF SCIENCES
DIETARY REFERENCE INTAKES:
ESTIMATED AVERAGE REQUIREMENTS

Life Stage Group	Phosphorus (mg/d)	Magnesium (mg/d)	Thiamin (mg/d)	Riboflavin (mg/d)	Niacin (mg/d)[a]
Children					
1–3 y	380	65	0.4	0.4	5
4–8 y	405	110	0.5	0.5	6
Males					
9–13 y	1,055	200	0.7	0.8	9
14–18 y	1,055	340	1.0	1.1	12
19–30 y	580	330	1.0	1.1	12
31–50 y	580	350	1.0	1.1	12
51–70 y	580	350	1.0	1.1	12
> 70 y	580	350	1.0	1.1	12
Females					
9–13 y	1,055	200	0.7	0.8	9
14–18 y	1,055	300	0.9	0.9	11
19–30 y	580	255	0.9	0.9	11
31–50 y	580	265	0.9	0.9	11
51–70 y	580	265	0.9	0.9	11
> 70 y	580	265	0.9	0.9	11
Pregnancy					
≤ 18 y	1,055	335	1.2	1.2	14
19–30 y	580	290	1.2	1.2	14
31–50 y	580	300	1.2	1.2	14
Lactation					
≤ 18 y	1,055	300	1.2	1.3	13
19–30 y	580	255	1.2	1.3	13
31–50 y	580	265	1.2	1.3	13

NOTE: This table presents Estimated Average Requirements (EARs), which serve two purposes: for assessing adequacy of population intakes, and as the basis for calculating Recommended Dietary Allowances (RDAs) for individuals for those nutrients. EARs have not been established for calcium, vitamin D, fluoride, pantothenic acid, biotin, or choline, or other nutrients not yet evaluated via the Dietary Reference Intake (DRI) process.

[a] As niacin equivalents (NE). 1 mg of niacin = 60 mg of tryptophan.

[b] As dietary folate equivalents (DFE). 1 DFE = 1 µg food folate = 0.6 µg of folic acid from fortified food or as a supplement consumed with food = 0.5 µg of a supplement taken on an empty stomach.

Vitamin B_6 (mg/d)	Folate (μg/d)[b]	Vitamin B_{12} (μg/d)	Vitamin C (mg/d)	Vitamin E (mg/d)[c]	Selenium (μg/d)
0.4	120	0.7	13	5	17
0.5	160	1.0	22	6	23
0.8	250	1.5	39	9	35
1.1	330	2.0	63	12	45
1.1	320	2.0	75	12	45
1.1	320	2.0	75	12	45
1.4	320	2.0	75	12	45
1.4	320	2.0	75	12	45
0.8	250	1.5	39	9	35
1.0	330	2.0	56	12	45
1.1	320	2.0	60	12	45
1.1	320	2.0	60	12	45
1.3	320	2.0	60	12	45
1.3	320	2.0	60	12	45
1.6	520	2.2	66	12	49
1.6	520	2.2	70	12	49
1.6	520	2.2	70	12	49
1.7	450	2.4	96	16	59
1.7	450	2.4	100	16	59
1.7	450	2.4	100	16	59

[c] As α-tocopherol. α-Tocopherol includes *RRR*-α-tocopherol, the only form of α-tocopherol that occurs naturally in foods, and the *2R*-stereoisomeric forms of α-tocopherol (*RRR*-, *RSR*-, *RRS*-, and *RSS*-α-tocopherol) that occur in fortified foods and supplements. It does not include the *2S*-stereoisomeric forms of α-tocopherol (*SRR*-, *SSR*-, *SRS*-, and *SSS*-α-tocopherol), also found in fortified foods and supplements.

FOOD AND NUTRITION BOARD, INSTITUTE OF MEDICINE— NATIONAL ACADEMY OF SCIENCES DIETARY REFERENCE INTAKES: TOLERABLE UPPER INTAKE LEVELS (UL[a])

Life Stage Group	Calcium (g/d)	Phosphorus (g/d)	Magnesium (mg/d)[b]	Vitamin D (μg/d)	Fluoride (mg/d)
Infants					
0–6 mo	ND[e]	ND	ND	25	0.7
7–12 mo	ND	ND	ND	25	0.9
Children					
1–3 y	2.5	3	65	50	1.3
4–8 y	2.5	3	110	50	2.2
Males, Females					
9–13 y	2.5	4	350	50	10
14–18 y	2.5	4	350	50	10
19–70 y	2.5	4	350	50	10
> 70 y	2.5	3	350	50	10
Pregnancy					
≤ 18 y	2.5	3.5	350	50	10
19–50 y	2.5	3.5	350	50	10
Lactation					
≤ 18 y	2.5	4	350	50	10
19–50 y	2.5	4	350	50	10

[a] UL = The maximum level of daily nutrient intake that is likely to pose no risk of adverse effects. Unless otherwise specified, the UL represents total intake from food, water, and supplements. Due to lack of suitable data, ULs could not be established for thiamin, riboflavin, vitamin B_{12}, pantothenic acid, biotin, or any carotenoids. In the absence of ULs, extra caution may be warranted in consuming levels above recommended intakes.

[b] The ULs for magnesium represent intake from a pharmacological agent only and do not include intake from food and water.

284

Niacin (mg/d)[c]	Vitamin B$_6$ (mg/d)	Folate (µg/d)[c]	Choline (g/d)	Vitamin C (mg/d)	Vitamin E (mg/d)[d]	Selenium (µg/d)
ND	ND	ND	ND	ND	ND	45
ND	ND	ND	ND	ND	ND	60
10	30	300	1.0	400	200	90
15	40	400	1.0	650	300	150
20	60	600	2.0	1,200	600	280
30	80	800	3.0	1,800	800	400
35	100	1,000	3.5	2,000	1,000	400
35	100	1,000	3.5	2,000	1,000	400
30	80	800	3.0	1,800	800	400
35	100	1,000	3.5	2,000	1,000	400
30	80	800	3.0	1,800	800	400
35	100	1,000	3.5	2,000	1,000	400

[c] The ULs for niacin, folate, and vitamin E apply to synthetic forms obtained from supplements, fortified foods, or a combination of the two.

[d] As α-tocopherol; applies to any form of supplemental α-tocopherol.

[e] ND = Not determinable due to lack of data of adverse effects in this age group and concern with regard to lack of ability to handle excess amounts. Source of intake should be from food only to prevent high levels of intake.